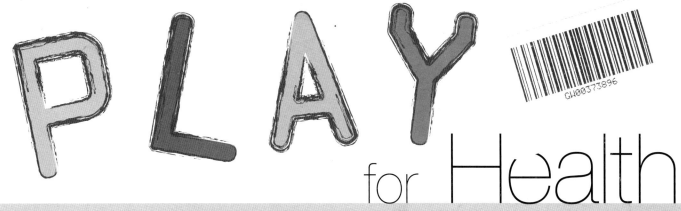

PLAY for Health

Delivering and Auditing Quality in Hospital Play Services

Judy Walker
BH(Hons) Reg HPSET

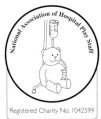

Registered Charity No. 1042599

National Association of Hospital Play Staff

Published 2006 by National Association of Hospital Play staff

Reg. Charity No 1042599

Coram Family, Coram Community Campus, 49
Mecklenburgh Square, London WC1N 2QA

www.nahps.org.uk

Copyright©National Association of Hospital Play Staff

NAHPS was founded in 1975 and became a registered
charity in 1992. Its charitable objects include the "promotion
of the physical and mental well being of children and young
people who are patients in hospital, hospice or receiving
medical care at home, by the promotion of high professional
standards for play staff, to ensure the provision of
appropriate therapeutic and stimulating play facilities and that
support is available to those who carry out this work."

ISBN- 13: 978-0-9554112-0-5

ISBN- 10: 0-9554112-0-3

Designed by Paul Burton

Printed by Wayzgoose

Acknowledgements

I would like to thank Peg Belson, Jackie McClelland, Nic Philips, Jean Wilde and Dr Richard Wilson for their support and advice during the development of this publication.

Contents

Section 3

Foreword

I am delighted to introduce this new publication from the National Association of Hospital Play Staff. We often tend to concentrate on delivering direct healthcare to children in hospitals when we should be considering the wider context in which that healthcare is delivered. The National Service Framework has been very clear about making services child friendly and that providing play specialists and play programmes are crucial elements for children in hospital. We have come a long way since the old days of barren environments for children in hospital and it would be a tragedy if we were now to allow services to step backwards because of lack of good provision and challenges on funding and resources.

This document is admirable not only in its purpose but also in the clear way in which it is set out. Hospital Trust boards, chief executives, managers and clinical staff will be able to see how they should be delivering quality in hospital play services and how they should audit what they are providing. It is a challenge for every Trust to audit its current provision, to see where it is falling short and to rectify those omissions. This document will help clinicians and managers to do exactly that. The Healthcare Commission has been important in inspecting services for children and previous inspections revealed that many hospitals were not good at providing child friendly environments or in promoting play services. I hope very much that use of this document will help to show a dramatic improvement next time the Healthcare Commission looks at these services within hospitals.

The contributors and editors, as well as the National Association of Hospital Play Staff, are to be congratulated on producing this important document, and paediatricians and nurses will welcome it and use it to further improve services for children.

Patricia Hamilton

Dr Patricia Hamilton
President
Royal College of Paediatrics and Child Health

SECTION

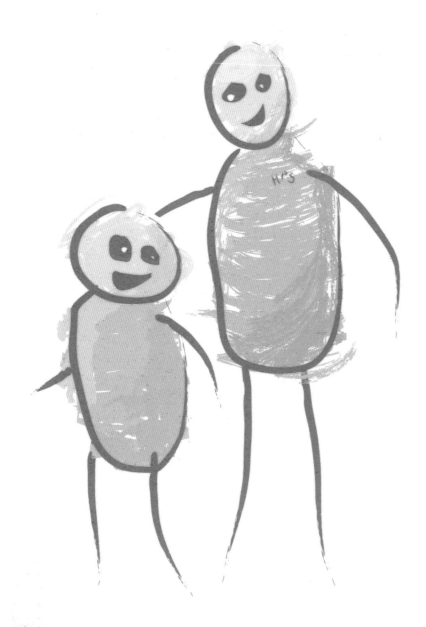

1

Introduction

"…unless we are making progress every year, month, every week, take my word for it we are going back" Florence Nightingale[1]

…unless we are making progress every year, month, every week, take my word for it we are going back

Florence Nightingale[1]

Those who provide and manage play services for child patients can do well to make Nightgale's statement their own and address the issue of "making progress" seriously. Free from the constraints of a national curriculum or rigorous OFSTED inspections, enriched by a workforce with a wonderful wealth of diverse backgrounds and knowledge and experience and operating within settings where goodwill is commonly flowing, progress is our obligation.

"Play for Health: Delivering and Auditing Quality in Hospital Play Services" is the successor to "Quality Management for Children: Play in Hospital"[2], published by the Play in Hospital Liaison Committee in 1990. This new document defines quality in hospital play services in a more structured format and includes areas of work not previously covered. Children's health services have been influenced by the publication of the National Service Framework for Children, Young People and Maternity Services[3] and the Government's White Paper "Every Child Matters"[4]. The hospital play specialist profession has evolved since 1990, with the numbers of hospital play specialists employed by the NHS increasing to an estimated 1,200. The proportion of qualified play specialists is growing rapidly. Hospital play is now a recognised and valued element of children's health services at every level.

In this new health service environment, the National Association of Hospital Play Staff (N.A.H.P.S) recognised the need to provide a tool to lead and guide the management and delivery of hospital play services over the next decade and beyond and commissioned this publication.

This audit tool uses Donabedian's Structure-Process-Outcome (SPO)[5] model, which was chosen after thorough research into a range of clinical audit tools. This model has a long history and has been used in a wide variety of settings and allows for all the issues relating to a particular topic to be clearly described, which benchmarking tools such as "Essence of Care"[6] do not. Hospital play services exist within structures which improve or restrict their functioning. These must be understood when assessing quality. Similarly, the actions or processes engaged in by play specialists are crucial factors in effective play service delivery.

The standards set in this document have their origins in a wide variety of publications and research. The author has also drawn on her 22 years of professional and managerial experience working as a hospital play specialist and during 17 years on the National Executive Committee of the National Association of Hospital Play Staff (N.A.H.P.S). Extensive consultation and dialogue also took place with senior professionals from the health service who have considerable experience of hospital play services

Classification of areas for audit

While few hospitals have the facilities to care for the three age groups described in this audit tool in separate areas, the roots of the British hospital play profession lie in psychodynamic and educational traditions, which recognise the differences between infancy, childhood and adolescence. This developmental approach is at the core of the work of the play specialist. Whilst an individual child may not easily fit into one developmental category (for example a teenager with delayed development), managers of play services must adopt a broad-brush approach and consider the needs of the majority.

The National Service Framework for Children and Young People[3] states that the differing needs of adolescents should to be recognised and met. As a result, we are witnessing a growth in the number of dedicated facilities for young people in hospital.

Standards for three different hospital settings have also been described in this publication. No distinction is made between the age groups of patients seen in these settings. The goals of hospital play services in these settings reflect the needs of the age groups, but it is the challenges posed by the settings that provide the audit material here. Some cross referencing of criteria may be required if, for example, there are babies on the paediatric unit, or young people seen in community settings.

While there are similarities between these chapters, most notably around risk management, documentation and training, dividing the six chapters in this way enables audit of specific areas or developmental groups.

Professional title

The professional title "play specialist" is used in this publication as it is in the National Service Framework for Children and Young People[3] and refers to a qualified hospital play specialist, registered with the Hospital Play Staff Education Trust (H.P.S.E.T.). Untrained staff can carry out some playroom tasks with direction and supervision, but the majority of processes described in this document require staff with the recognised professional training and suitable clinical experience.

While the inclusion of the word "play" in the job title suggests innocence and simplicity, the need to ensure that the public are given the very highest standard of care and protected from people untrained for the role, is as necessary in hospital play services as in any other work with children.

An overview of the functions of hospital play

The National Service Framework for Children and Young People[3] provides clear guidance on the provision of play services throughout the NHS. Many previous publications [7-12] have also endorsed the provision of hospital play services. The 2005/06 Healthcare Commission Self Assessment Framework Improvement Review for children's services includes criteria to assess the provision of play services and the employment of play specialists. Inclusion in this audit has consolidated official recognition of the value of hospital play programmes.

There is ample theoretical and empirical evidence on the functions of play in childhood. Under normal circumstances the lives of infants, children and young people will be dominated by their play, through which they develop physical, cognitive, emotional and psychosocial skills. This one issue, the need to play in hospital settings to ensure normal development continues, should alone be enough to explain the necessity of providing of play programmes for in-patient children.

The hospital experience, whether it is as an in- or out-patient, presents the child or young person with a very particular challenge. Separation from much that is familiar such as family members, domestic routines and the safety of the home environment, can be experienced as anything from mildly disorientating to catastrophic depending on the individual concerned. Added to that the introduction of a whole new environment where unpredictable events occur, a large number of new adults are encountered and many new experiences are had one after another and it is common to find high levels of anxiety. These events are happening at a time when the child is likely to be at their most vulnerable being ill, injured or requiring surgery, and when their main carers are also worried and anxious.

Play has a simple but vital function of introducing the familiar to the unfamiliarity of the hospital setting. The provision of play equipment in itself will signal directly to the child "children are welcome here". The hospital environment is full of new sights, frightening equipment, large machines or sick adults, so the sight of favourite and appealing toys is welcome and reassuring. Children and young people may feel unsure of the correct way to behave in hospital or what they should do, but they know how to play and engage willingly in it if given encouragement. These opportunities to participate in play on their own, or with other children, encourage adaptation and adjustment.

For patients who have experienced trauma or upset or have had surgery, play activities encourage them to regain confidence in their abilities and their bodies and can contribute to physiotherapy and occupational therapy goals. Parents also benefit from this normative function of play as they observe their children at play and receive a message of reassurance at the sight of the involved in playful activity.

For babies, the hospital represents a deprived environment in terms of stimulating sensory experiences to support their developmental progress. Guided play activity enriches the opportunities for beneficial, pleasurable and satisfying sensory experiences and can help redress the imbalance of pain and discomfort sensations caused by medical interventions.

Valuable information can be gathered to inform the child's care and treatment from observation of children at play, such as the type of play engaged in, whether or not the child can settle to play, whether pain is forgotten during play as well as themes emerging in their creative or imaginative play and interactions with adults. Play is a language that children use to think for themselves as well as communicate with others and the play specialist is mindful of this in the facilitation of play opportunities for even the sickest child.

Directed play to enable the child to communicate with the team on specific topics, especially around choice and consent, is another example of how play acts as a communication bridge between adult carers and the child. The young patient has a right to have his or her views and questions about treatment to be heard[13] but they are less likely to be able to be able to express those views. Play can be the medium through which those views can be spoken and heard. Many children and young people will have fears and misconceptions about what might happen to them in hospital. For some these will be minor and manageable within their own cognitive and emotional reasoning processes. For others, anxiety may not be manageable and directed and non-directed play allows for these to be expressed, explored and understood.

With guidance from play specialists, play is the tool through which children in hospital can move beyond an everyday understanding of their experience. Just as a child can be helped to make sense of numerical concepts through play with a school teacher so too can s/he be helped to develop new knowledge with the intervention of the play specialist. The hospital presents a different "cultural form" and provides the child with rich learning opportunities.

Some of the functions of play in the hospital setting described here also apply to psychotherapy, but hospital play is not play therapy. Hospital play relates to experiences in the present. Its aim is to minimise negative reactions to being in hospital. On the whole, children seen by play specialists are healthy, stable children who have been temporarily placed in an abnormally stressful situation. The reduction of anxiety levels together with the many other benefits associated with the provision of play can be experienced as therapeutic.

The communicative function of play combines as both as a learning tool for children and a means of addressing specific fears and misconceptions in what is called "play preparation". Structured play to introduce developmentally appropriate information about forthcoming procedures has a strong research base[14-25] which demonstrates its effectiveness in reducing anxiety and increasing co-operative behaviours. There is also evidence that it can reduce negative physical after effects of surgery. By replacing fantasies with facts and encouraging and rehearsing helpful coping skills, the child enters the anaesthetic room or treatment room prepared both cognitively and emotionally for the experience having done the "work of worrying"[26] in the playroom.

Play preparation for procedures needs to be designed to suit the individual child and their circumstances and timed according to the situation. Several sessions, and a home visit may be required for a young child facing a complex operation or a long course of radiotherapy treatment. While other hospital staff and parents can and do prepare children for their treatment experiences, or distract them during them, the play specialist has this as his or her primary role and will ensure the necessary support is provided.

Distraction play provides an alternative focus during medical procedures, and can reduce pain responses. The presence of the play specialist to perform alternative focus activities enables paediatric staff to complete their task, causing the minimum distress to the child and family.

The provision of play equipment is not alone enough to ensure play occurs in hospital. Anxious and sick children are less likely to engage in play than their well peers and may need very specific help to do so if they have restrictions on their movement or position. In a detailed age related study of the social functions of play in hospital, it was found that the presence of an adult is imperative if the child is to engage in play and thus resume normal functional behaviour.[27]

While all paediatric staff can use play in their care of the child, the play specialist holds the responsibility for ensuring the essential functions of play described above are built into the fabric of the child's journey through the hospital experience.

The organisation and management of hospital play services

Those holding the recognised professional training referred to in this publication need also to be registered with the Hospital Play Staff Education Trust (H.P.S.E.T.) and ensure they renew that registration every five years with evidence of continuing professional development activities. This training has been in place since 1975 and became a nationally standardised accredited qualification under BTEC Edexcel in 1985. In 2005, the NVQ Level 4 Professional Development Diploma in Specialised Play for Sick Children and Young People was introduced. At this time, the NVQ level 3 was phased out.

There are three main organisational models for hospital play services operating in the UK. The number of play specialists employed in the hospital or Trust largely dictates which model is used.

A "play co-ordinator "or "play services manager", that is, someone who is a qualified play specialist and has additional training in staff management and leadership, often manages large teams of play specialists. Depending on staff numbers, the "play co-ordinator" or "play services manager" may or may not work on the ward. For teams of eight staff and upwards, it is likely that the play co-ordinator will not have day-to-day responsibility for the ward playroom although he/she may carry a caseload of patients with complex needs. The budget for play specialist salaries is most often part of the ward staff budget. When a play co-ordinator is employed, it is more likely that this will be managed centrally. Some hospitals have a mix of styles, as some wards prefer to hold on to their "own" play specialist budget, while others prefer to have it managed by the play manager.

The second model sees the provision of specialist play services, such as preparation for surgery and therapeutic needle play, managed centrally on a referral basis. Ward based playrooms are staffed by play assistants or trainee play specialists, while the specialised activities of the hospital play specialists are managed by a play co-ordinator.

The third model is often seen in smaller paediatric teams, where the ward sister or modern matron manages two or three play specialists in one hospital. Paediatric nurses are often the best advocates for play services for children in hospital and are trained staff managers. They are not however, qualified play specialists and this can lead to a shortfall when professional guidance is required or advice is sought. By participating in the growing numbers of local professional networks and attending national conferences, play specialists can access useful support and guidance. For lone or small groups of play specialists managed by nurses, there is a concern that standards and motivation to maintain and improve services will slip.

The nature of play specialist work, where they usually run their own ward based playroom and see other play specialists only occasionally, and are out numbered by the majority of other staff groups, means there are particular benefits to organising staff within a hospital or trust under a single qualified play specialist. The quality of the services provided, the proficiency of the play specialists' work and the maintenance of professional boundaries will be enhanced with the appropriate leadership and management. The NHS Management Executive (1992)[28] supported this and described the "material improvements in the quality of care of drawing play specialists into a single cohesive group".

Using this Book

To improve the quality of play services we first have to understand the service inside and out. Without knowledge of the structures, processes and outcomes of current services, "improvements" may be inappropriate, unsustainable or ineffective.

Audit is a broad term which describes the process of gathering information to inform the quality improvement process. Audit is part of a circular journey where knowledge gained is used to make improvements which are then assessed to see the benefits that have resulted and if any further adjustments should be made.

Quality is created in hospital play services by the structures, (facilities, human resources and organisational characteristics) processes (the activities and decisions undertaken by staff and patients to achieve specified objectives) and outcomes (changes in health status, knowledge, behaviour and satisfaction of patients).

Assessment of these factors helps to define quality. The aim here is to create clear and measurable criteria for the structures, processes and outcomes at the core of hospital play services.

While this publication lists the criteria to guide you in audit, it does not define assessment methods. These will depend on the resources for audit and the subject you are auditing. The audit tool itself can be used in a variety of ways. For example, it is possible to audit by structures alone, or by choosing a number of specific outcomes or processes and comparing these across settings (see Appendix). The advantage of separating the criteria is that if an outcome is not achieved, the structures and processes necessary have already been identified and therefore the source of the problem is clear. Cause and effect between structures, processes and outcomes is not linear and indeed is often quite complex. The numerical system used does not link across structures, processes and outcomes.

The audit cycle should involve;

1. Defining best practice. Many audit cycles begin with a review of the available evidence on the chosen topic. This may include a literature search, visits to other services, the gathering of national and local clinical guidelines and policies, the use of professional expertise and incorporation of the preferences of services users. The chapters in this publication outline best practice in three settings and for three different age groups but further evidence of best practice can be gathered.

2. Deciding what to audit. Given the time and energy involved, it is important to have a clear reason for carrying out an audit, as well as commitment to the quality improvement process. Possible reasons include:

- **poor** performance
- **poor** results in a patient satisfaction survey
- **to highlight** good practice in one department
- **to develop** an understanding of an issue across a region
- **to contribute** to national assessment frameworks or targets
- **to address** a serious adverse incident report
- **to improve** services for patients
- **to increase** the efficiency of play services
- **to increase** the safety of play services
- **to improve** staff recruitment and retention

3. Involving the right people at the start. Gathering together a team of staff committed to the quality improvement process will greatly improve your chances of success. The more staff that are involved, the more widespread the dissemination of good practice will be. In fact, numerous audits of documentation by nurses have shown that the quality and quantity of documentation improved as soon as an audit group was set up and before the audit had actually taken place!

4. Gathering and measuring the evidence. There are a number of examples of how you might go about auditing aspects of your service using the Structure Process Outcome model provided the Appendix of this publication. This stage is the heart of the quality improvement process and should not be undertaken in isolation.

5. Taking action where necessary. The audit itself is just the start of the improvement process. As previously stated, improvements often start as soon as the audit group is set up; the staff team focuses on the issue to be audited. By involving staff at different

grades and from different disciplines, awareness of the subject will increase. The audit itself may yield positive results that should be publicised and acknowledged appropriately. However, if analysis of the audit results reveals poor standards, audit group must discuss these fully. The Structure Process Outcome model will help problem solving and give pointers as to how the quality of services can be improved. The audit team will need to decide how to action solutions in each individual setting. In a large hospital trust with a good training budget, solutions may differ to those in a small paediatric unit with no training budget.

6.Implementing change. Prepare an action plan and put in place changes to improve the quality of the play service. Allow a period of time for the changes to take effect.

7.Re-auditing. In order to establish whether the changes implemented have been effective, it is necessary to re–audit after a suitable period of time. Rapid changes in service configuration may mean that some adjustments have to be made to your original audit methods. To reinforce the value of the quality improvement process undertaken, and increase its chances of being sustainable, publicity and promotion through internal and external media should take place.

SECTION

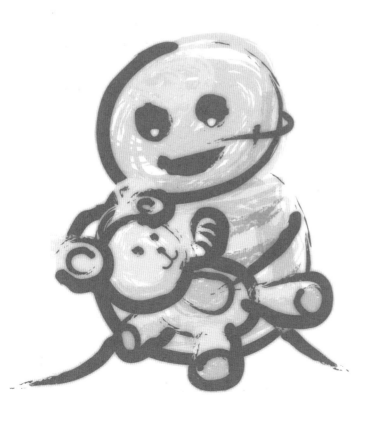

2

Paediatric In-patients

PAEDIATRIC IN-PATIENTS

SUB TOPIC   **CREATION AND MAINTENANCE OF AN AGE APPROPRIATE ENVIRONMENT**

CARE GROUP   All children on the paediatric ward

STANDARD

OBJECTIVE   To create and maintain an environment where children can access play activities suitable to their developmental abilities. To ensure that health and safety guidelines are complied with.

RATIONALE   Play is a basic requirement for normal, healthy development. Without supervised play services, children's play opportunities will be limited and normal development restricted. Where there is no structured play service, the number of adverse incidents is likely to increase.

STRUCTURES   S1 Playrooms are close to patient bed areas enabling patients to participate in play within reach of medical, nursing and parental care.

S2 The size and layout of the play environment allows parents/carers and staff to participate in play activities.

S3 Adequate storage facilities for play equipment are provided. Space is available for the maintenance and cleaning of this equipment and the play areas.

S4 Play specialists receive training and guidance on risk management practices including infection control, use of electrical equipment, storage, theft, damage, internet access and manual handling.

S5 The requirements of children with restricted mobility, sensory impairment and/or special needs are taken into account in the design and funding of play environments.

S6 Ward managers, modern matrons and play specialists have mechanisms in place for liaison regarding play environments.

S7 Sufficient funding is allocated to allow the periodic review and renewal of play equipment.

S8 New play specialists, volunteers and students are provided with written information about risk management practices for play environments.

S9 The play environment is culturally inclusive. Play materials, books, music and equipment appropriate to the age, development, gender, ethnicity, physical restrictions and sensory impairments of patients are provided.

PAEDIATRIC IN-PATIENTS

SUB TOPIC cont.	**CREATION AND MAINTENANCE OF AN AGE APPROPRIATE ENVIRONMENT**
PROCESSES	P1 Play specialists store toys and games so that the necessary room cleaning can take place.
	P2 Play specialists organise and set out a range of play activities depending on their assessment of patient needs, the seasonal and religious calendar and staffing ratios.
	P3 Play specialists maintain an awareness of new play products and involve patients in the planning for new purchases and any changes.
	P4 Play specialists provide recreational equipment that is suitable for early, middle and late childhood, and that reflects a diversity of cultures and physical and intellectual abilities.
	P5 Play specialists ensure regular washing of toys and equipment used by children takes place in line with local infection control policies.
OUTCOMES	O1 All children are able to engage in play activities daily, exercising choice in a safe and clean environment.
	O2 Parents/carers and members of staff can use the play environment and demonstrate respect for the activities and equipment within it.
	O3 Risks in designated play areas are minimised.
SUB TOPIC	**PROVISION OF RECREATIONAL AND THERAPEUTIC PLAY ACTIVITIES**
CARE GROUP	Patients over 2 years of age nursed on the paediatric ward
STANDARD	
OBJECTIVE	Patients are provided with a range of play activities to promote their motor, social, cognitive and emotional development, and encourage adaptation to the hospital environment. These will contribute to the medical and nursing objectives and promote emotional health.
RATIONALE	The hospitalised child is emotionally and developmentally vulnerable. Recreational and therapeutic play activities provide opportunities for reflective and mastery play, and interaction with other children.
STRUCTURES	S1 Play specialists are employed in sufficient numbers to provide play activities for the majority of the day and to ensure equality of access is maintained.
	S2 Each paediatric in-patient unit has a playroom with sufficient space to accommodate a wide variety of play activities.

PAEDIATRIC IN-PATIENTS

SUB TOPIC cont. **PROVISION OF RECREATIONAL AND THERAPEUTIC PLAY ACTIVITIES**

STRUCTURES

S3 Sufficient storage space is allocated for the safe storage of play equipment.

S4 Access arrangements to the ward playroom are agreed between the play specialist and the ward manager. Patient safety is maintained.

S5 Patients with restricted mobility are given equal access to activity programmes.

S6 Play specialists receive daily handovers from nursing staff.

S7 Care plans include recognition of the need to play, and contributions from play specialists.

S8 Sufficient funds are provided to purchase safe and appropriate toys, games, craft materials and large play equipment.

PROCESSES

P1 Play specialists introduce all new patients and their carers to the play programme.

P2 Play specialists assess the needs, abilities and interests of each patient, and set short and long-term goals.

P3 Play specialists liaise with the multi-professional team and family members to arrange times for play sessions.

P4 Leadership, interaction and support during play is provided, where appropriate. Non-directive play, free of adult intervention, takes place.

P5 Parents/carers are encouraged to be involved in play activities and are kept informed of the play specialist assessments and plans.

P6 Play specialists create and maintain an environment where satisfying and spontaneous play takes place.

P7 Play specialists observe children at play noting themes, physical abilities, and interactions with real and/or imaginary people.

P8 Play specialists praise the endeavours of patients, enhancing their self esteem.

P9 Play specialists document patient names, ages and the type of play services used for clinical governance purposes.

OUTCOMES

O1 Each child is able to participate in a range of play activities, as fully as he/she wishes or is able.

O2 Parents/carers have access to suitable play equipment.

O3 Play opportunities which meet the developmental, adaptation and emotional needs of individual patients are provided.

SUB TOPIC Cont. **PROVISION OF RECREATIONAL AND THERAPEUTIC PLAY ACTIVITIES**

OUTCOMES

O4 Patients and their families are aware of the role of the play specialist, the play service hours and the importance of play in hospital.

O5 Assessments, interventions and evaluations undertaken by the play specialist are documented in the patient care plan or notes.

O6 All professionals caring for the child are able to access information about play activities and needs.

O7 Play service numerical data is collated and published periodically.

SUB TOPIC **ACTIVITIES TO PROMOTE AND SUSTAIN NORMAL GROWTH AND DEVELOPMENT**

CARE GROUP

Patients over 2 years of age nursed on the paediatric ward

STANDARD

OBJECTIVE

To ensure developmental progress is maintained and opportunities for learning are maximised during a hospital admission.

RATIONALE

Lengthy and/or repeated hospital admissions, can lead to developmental delay. Individual developmental play programmes can be developed to address this issue.

STRUCTURES

S1 The play specialist team includes experienced members of staff who can lead and guide developmental play programmes.

S2 The requirements for developmentally stimulating play for children with a range of abilities are considered when purchasing equipment and setting budgets.

S3 Play specialists meet regularly with members of the multi-disciplinary team (teachers, physiotherapists, speech and language therapists and occupational therapists) to discuss the developmental needs of patients.

S4 Play specialists contribute to the shared documentation for each patient.

PROCESSES

P1 Play specialists observe and assess the developmental progress of long term patients and those who have repeated admissions.

P2 Structured play programmes are created for individual children.

P3 Children are able to participate in construction, imaginary, physical and sensory play and social interaction.

P4 Play specialists adapt play activities for patients who have restricted movement and/or special needs.

PAEDIATRIC IN-PATIENTS

SUB TOPIC Cont. | **ACTIVITIES TO PROMOTE AND SUSTAIN NORMAL GROWTH AND DEVELOPMENT**

PROCESSES | P5 Play specialists build on the child's knowledge of hospitalisation and encourage the development and articulation of their understanding using a variety of approaches.

OUTCOMES | O1 Children's hospital experiences include a wide range of enjoyable, developmentally stimulating play activities.

O2 All patients have access to the benefits of play activities.

O3 Children are helped to use the unique learning opportunities provided by the hospital setting.

SUB TOPIC | **MAINTAINING LINKS WITH HOME AND FAMILIAR ROUTINES**

CARE GROUP | All patients especially those who have an extended stay in hospital

STANDARD |

OBJECTIVE | To ensure that children in hospital maintain links with home and family routines. To reassure children about the continuity of home life and their place in it through play activities provided by play specialists. To acknowledge cultural diversity.

RATIONALE | The hospitalised child is separated from family life and familiar routines. Engagement in play activities directed at maintaining links with home ensures that the child keeps the subject of normal family life to the fore. Concerns and misunderstandings, identified through play can be addressed.

STRUCTURES | S1 Care plans include the need to maintain familiar routines and contributions from play specialists.

S2 Play specialists are able to allocate sufficient time to carry out this aspect of care.

S3 Play specialists promote awareness of separation issues within the multi-disciplinary team.

S4 Play specialists attend training on diversity and spirituality.

PROCESSES | P1 The play specialist uses a variety of play activities to enable the child to maintain links family, friends and home.

P2 The play specialist acknowledges the significance of the personal belongings, preferences and routines of the patient through play activities and dialogue.

P3 The play specialist gathers information about and respects family routines and preferences.

PAEDIATRIC IN-PATIENTS

SUB TOPIC Cont.   **MAINTAINING LINKS WITH HOME AND FAMILIAR ROUTINES**

PROCESSES

P4 The play specialist involves parents/carers in play activities.

P5 The play specialist regularly engages the child and family in discussions about family and home.

P6 The play specialist acknowledges issues around separation from siblings, extended family, pets and friends in discussions and play activities.

P7 The play specialist recognises anticipatory anxiety and encourages adaptation in preparation for discharge home.

OUTCOMES

O1 Maladaptive behaviours associated with separation from home and family are minimised.

O2 The child retains his identity in the family.

O3 Parental and patient anxiety before and after discharge home is minimised.

SUB TOPIC   **PRE-ADMISSION INFORMATION AND SUPPORT**

CARE GROUP

Patients and their families due to be admitted to the paediatric in-patient ward

STANDARD

OBJECTIVE

To provide accessible and meaningful information for children and their families prior to admission.

RATIONALE

Children are prone to misconceptions and anxieties about hospital admissions. Information designed specifically for children and young people is essential.

STRUCTURES

S1 Information provision is part of the clinical governance requirements of the paediatric unit.

S2 Play specialists are aware of the processes for consultation, advice and approval of written information for patients and their families.

S3 Internet pages, booklets, videos, photographs and/or information sheets are produced specifically for paediatric patients and their families.

S4 Funding and equipment resources are available to play specialists developing information materials.

S5 Play specialists are able to allocate time to the development of information materials.

S6 Mechanisms exist for the translation of information materials into languages reflecting the ethnicity of the local population.

PAEDIATRIC IN-PATIENTS

SUB TOPIC Cont.   **MAINTAINING LINKS WITH HOME AND FAMILIAR ROUTINES**

PROCESSES   P1 Patients and their families are consulted about the content of information written by play specialists, which is reviewed and approved by other paediatric staff prior to use.

P2 The source of all information provided by play specialists is clearly identified and dated.

P3 Effective means of delivering appropriate information are identified through training, consultation and research.

P4 Patients and their families are consulted when developing information materials.

P5 Audits are undertaken to evaluate the uptake of information by patients and their families.

OUTCOMES   O1 All patients and their families receive timely, meaningful information prior to their admission to hospital.

O2 Patients and their families are able to seek further support and information if they so wish.

SUB TOPIC   **PREPARATION FOR INVESTIGATIONS, SURGERY AND MEDICAL PROCEDURES**

CARE GROUP   Children aged 2 to 12 years

STANDARD

OBJECTIVE   Patients are able to understand, at a developmentally appropriate level, the procedure they are to experience. To enable patients to develop adaptive coping strategies. To enable patients to participate in the consent process.

RATIONALE   The UN Convention on the Rights of the Child states that the child has the right to be fully involved in decisions about his care. A child centred approach to information giving enables children's participation in the consent process.

Research has demonstrated that preparation through play reduces anxiety, supports effective pain management and encourages co-operative behaviour.

STRUCTURES   S1 Play specialist hours of employment enable them to assess, plan and implement preparation programmes when required.

S2 Paediatric units have mechanisms in place to ensure play specialists are informed of planned procedures.

PAEDIATRIC IN-PATIENTS

SUB TOPIC Cont. **PREPARATION FOR INVESTIGATIONS, SURGERY AND MEDICAL PROCEDURES**

STRUCTURES

S3 Play specialists undertake ongoing education to ensure excellence in preparation techniques, including reflective practice, peer review, professional conferences and local teaching sessions.

S4 Preparation interventions are recorded in the appropriate documentation.

PROCESSES

P1 The play specialist gathers information about the patient requiring preparation through observation and interaction with the child and dialogue with family and staff members.

P2 Parents/carers are fully informed of the reasons for preparation and the approach to be taken.

P3 The play specialist assesses the child's psychological responses to learning. The play specialist provides verbal information and uses visual aids to prepare the child.

P4 The play specialist engages the child in preparation play, monitoring verbal and non-verbal communication throughout, in one or more sessions.

P5 The play specialist halts preparation play if the child shows undue anxiety, and explores the possible reasons for this anxiety at an appropriate time.

P6 The play specialist acknowledges anxiety about pain, and works collaboratively with staff and carers to address the child's concerns.

P7 The play specialist informs parents/carers of the outcomes of the play preparation and the coping strategies identified.

P8 The play specialist reports directly to the patient's nurse and documents the content and outcome of preparation.

P9 The play specialist returns to the patient to facilitate post procedural mastery play and debriefing.

OUTCOMES

O1 Age appropriate preparation for procedures, based on the circumstances of the individual, is carried out in a timely fashion.

O2 Parents/carers are informed of the purpose, content and outcome of preparation.

O3 The record of preparation is accessible to all health professionals involved with the child.

PAEDIATRIC IN-PATIENTS

SUB TOPIC	**POST- TREATMENT OR POST-PROCEDURAL PLAY**
CARE GROUP	Children aged 2 to 12 who have undergone invasive medical or surgical procedures or treatment
STANDARD	
OBJECTIVE	The play specialist ensures that children have the opportunity to achieve mastery and understanding of invasive treatment or procedures.
RATIONALE	Post-procedural play gives the child the opportunity to reflect on and make sense of hospital experiences. Achievements can be recognised and praised. Observations made during post-procedural play sessions can be incorporated into the care plan.
STRUCTURES	S1 Play specialists allocate time to see patients following invasive medical and surgical procedures.
	S2 Regular liaison with the multi-disciplinary team takes place. Post procedural play is planned, assessed and discussed.
	S3 Opportunities for clinical supervision and reflective practice are provided for play specialists to enable them to develop their knowledge and expertise in this field
PROCESSES	P1 The play specialist facilitates therapeutic post-procedural play in a safe environment providing a variety of materials through which children can engage in mastery play and communicate their concerns.
	P2 The play specialist gathers information about the child's experiences during the procedure from family and staff members.
	P3 Positive coping strategies and helpful behaviours are acknowledged and reinforced, either verbally or through reward certificates, stickers or other motivators.
	P4 The play specialist reassures parents if they are anxious about the child's emotional responses during a procedure.
	P5 The outcome of post-procedural play is shared with parents/carers. Advice and suggestions for ongoing support are given.
OUTCOMES	O1 Children's anxiety levels after procedures are reduced through the provision of supportive play opportunities.
	O2 Parents/carers feel able to help their child adjust after the hospital experience.

PAEDIATRIC IN-PATIENTS

SUB TOPIC Cont.   **POST- TREATMENT OR POST-PROCEDURAL PLAY**

OUTCOMES
   O3 Members of the multi-disciplinary team communicate effectively about post-procedural care. Patients with particular problems are referred on where necessary

   O4 The play specialist documents outcomes of post-procedural play in the child's notes.

SUB TOPIC   **DISTRACTION THERAPY AND ALTERNATIVE FOCUS ACTIVITIES**

CARE GROUP
   Children having medical procedures or investigations

STANDARD

OBJECTIVE
   Play specialists enable patients to cope with clinical procedures and investigations by providing an alternative focus for their attention

RATIONALE
   Distraction therapy and alternative focus activities help children to cope with procedures by diverting their attention. Children are therefore less likely to be distressed and non-compliant, which creates a safer clinical environment. Children can gain confidence in themselves and those who care for them. As a result of the distraction therapy, the child may experience less pain.

STRUCTURES
   S1 Play specialist hours of employment enable them to provide distraction therapy when required.

   S2 Paediatric units have mechanisms in place to ensure play specialists are informed of planned procedures.

   S3 Play specialists undertake ongoing education to ensure excellence in distraction techniques.

   S4 There is funding for distraction equipment.

   S5 The provision of distraction during procedures is an integral part of the holding still/restraint policy.

PROCESSES
   P1 The play specialist gathers information about the procedure and establishes a distraction therapy plan in conjunction with the team members involved.

   P2 When distracting older children, the distraction techniques to be used are discussed and, where appropriate and possible, rehearsed prior to the event.

   P3 If the play specialist is to be present to lead the distraction, the role he/she will play is explained to the family and team members involved.

PAEDIATRIC IN-PATIENTS

SUB TOPIC Cont.   **DISTRACTION THERAPY AND ALTERNATIVE FOCUS ACTIVITIES**

PROCESSES
P4 Where the play specialist is not going to accompany the child, he/she provides feedback to the staff and family members involved, and play equipment for distraction or alternative focus activities.

P5 The play specialist praises specific achievements and all positive coping behaviours demonstrated by the child and rewards with certificates and/or stickers, where appropriate.

P6 Distraction therapy techniques and outcomes are documented in the child's notes.

OUTCOMES
O1 Age appropriate distraction therapy based on the needs of the individual is carried out in a timely fashion.

O2 Parents/carers understand and support the distraction therapy.

O3 The child's experience of pain is reduced by the use of alternative focus activities.

O4 A record of the distraction therapy/alternative focus activity is accessible to all health professionals involved with the child.

SUB TOPIC   **THERAPEUTIC PLAY ACTIVITIES**

CARE GROUP
Children aged 2 to 12 years where there is a defined concern

STANDARD

OBJECTIVE
Issues which arise as a result of hospital experiences, illness or treatment are identified and responded to using a range of age appropriate therapeutic techniques.

RATIONALE
Illness and/or hospital experiences in childhood may cause short or long term psychological harm. Children who are identified as having increased anxieties are provided with additional support through therapeutic play sessions.

STRUCTURES
S1 The play specialist team includes staff with considerable experience who can lead and guide therapeutic play.

S2 The play specialist team work schedule is organised to permit flexibility for one-to-one therapeutic work.

S3 Play specialists have regular contact with members of the psychology team for clinical supervision for therapeutic work.

S4 Play specialists attend regular multi-professional team meetings where therapeutic work can be discussed and patients referred on if required.

PAEDIATRIC IN-PATIENTS

SUB TOPIC Cont.   **THERAPEUTIC PLAY ACTIVITIES**

PROCESSES

P1 The play specialist observes and assesses the child's verbal and non-verbal communication during play for atypical behaviour.

P2 Therapeutic play interventions are planned, implemented and evaluated within one or more in-patient admissions or on an out-patient basis.

P3 A variety of materials and approaches are used to initiate mastery play and the resolution of issues related to the hospital experience.

P4 The play specialist promotes the child's ability to make choices and feel in control of their experiences in liaison with family and multi-disciplinary team members.

P5 The play specialist discusses the goals of therapeutic play and observations made with parents/carers.

P6 The play specialist ensures the issues identified are documented and shared with key professionals in the child's life.

OUTCOMES

O1 Parents/carers are informed about therapeutic play activities.

O2 Children identified by the play specialist, parents/carers or members of the multi-disciplinary team, as having increased anxieties are provided with additional support through planned therapeutic play activities.

O3 Therapeutic play sessions are documented and available to all health professionals involved with the child.

SUB TOPIC   **PLAY FOR CHILDREN WHO HAVE RESTRICTED MOVEMENT**

CARE GROUP   Children aged 2 to 12 years

STANDARD

OBJECTIVE   Children with newly acquired or pre-existing restricted movement are able to participate fully in play activities whilst in hospital. Play specialists address their specific needs.

RATIONALE   Play is a familiar and satisfying activity, which has therapeutic and functional benefits for children who have restricted movement.

STRUCTURES

S1 Play specialists are employed in sufficient numbers to ensure that children with restricted movement have daily play sessions on a one-to-one basis.

S2 The play programme has a wide range of play equipment suitable for patients with restricted movement.

PAEDIATRIC IN-PATIENTS

SUB TOPIC Cont. **PLAY FOR CHILDREN WHO HAVE RESTRICTED MOVEMENT**

STRUCTURES
S3 Play specialists meet regularly with physiotherapists, occupational therapists and nurses to plan the care for children with restricted movement.

S4 The needs of children with restricted movement are included in play specialist training.

S5 Play specialists receive daily ward reports keeping them informed of the nursing care for children with restricted movement.

PROCESSES
P1 Play specialists enable children with restricted movement to access a wide range of play activities.

P2 Stimulating, social and therapeutic play encounters are facilitated by play specialists who demonstrate flexibility and imagination to ensure the child with restricted movement receives the full benefit of play in hospital.

P3 Parents/carers are encouraged to participate in playful activities with their children and are provided with toys and games.

P4 Where restricted movement is an outcome of trauma or hospital intervention, play specialists provide therapeutic play sessions to enable adjustment and adaptation.

OUTCOMES
O1 Children with restricted movement have equal access to play services.

O2 The risk of developmental delay and additional stress caused by restricted movement is minimised through regular supported play activities.

O3 The care received is coordinated between all members of the multi-disciplinary team.

O4 Written play programmes are passed to the community team when patients with newly acquired restricted movement are discharged.

PAEDIATRIC IN-PATIENTS

SUB TOPIC   **CHILDREN IN ISOLATION**

CARE GROUP
: All paediatric in-patients who require isolation due to reduced immunity, infectious conditions or radioactivity

STANDARD

OBJECTIVE
: To provide play programmes for children who require isolation. To provide sensory stimulation and social interaction to children in isolation. To address misconceptions and anxieties.

RATIONALE
: Children who require isolation due to reduced immunity, infectious conditions or radioactivity, have restricted play and social opportunities. This can hinder normal development. Play programmes can address misconceptions and anxieties and promote coping behaviours.

STRUCTURES
: S1 Play specialists are employed in sufficient numbers to ensure that children in isolation rooms have daily play sessions.

S2 Play service funding includes recognition of the additional resources required by isolation patients.

S3 All members of the multi-disciplinary team share information about children in isolation.

S4 Play specialists are allocated storage space for the play equipment required by patients in isolation.

S5 Play specialists receive training on infection control procedures and health and safety requirements relating directly to their work with isolation patients.

PROCESSES
: P1 Play specialists provide a wide range of stimulating play activities to meet the developmental needs of this group.

P2 Play specialists use play activities to address the effects of the restricted social environment and to maintain links with outside world.

P3 Play specialists enable parents/carers and members of staff to lead play activities in the isolation environment.

P4 Play specialists ensure that the cleaning, disposal and storage of play equipment for isolation patients is carried out according to established health and safety guidelines.

P5 Play programmes are prepared for long term isolation patients, which are accessible to family and team members. These are up-dated regularly.

PAEDIATRIC IN-PATIENTS

SUB TOPIC Cont. **CHILDREN IN ISOLATION**

OUTCOMES O1 Patients in isolation receive regular planned input from play specialists, which is geared to their individual needs.

O2 The developmental and psychological risks associated with isolating children are reduced through the implementation of play programmes.

O3 Health and safety policies and guidelines are adhered to.

SUB TOPIC **SUPPORT FOR GRIEF AND BEREAVEMENT ISSUES**

CARE GROUP Terminally ill children and their families, or those who have recently experienced a major loss. Children dealing with losses associated with illness and accidents.

STANDARD

OBJECTIVE Play specialists use play activities and their relationship with the child to informally and formally support children dealing with grief and bereavement issues.

RATIONALE Play is both a channel for communication and a means of processing difficult issues. Play specialists can actively support children with terminal illness or experiencing other major loss.

STRUCTURES S1 The play specialist team includes staff with considerable experience and training who can lead and guide work on grief and bereavement issues.

S2 The play specialist team work schedule is organised to permit flexibility for one-to-one bereavement work.

S3 Play specialists have regular contact with members of the psychology team for clinical supervision and supervision of bereavement work.

S4 Play specialists attend regular multi-professional team meetings where bereavement work can be discussed and patients referred on if required.

PROCESSES P1 The play specialist observes and assesses children's verbal and non-verbal communication during play for issues around grief and loss.

P2 The play specialist acknowledges the significance of the patient's feelings and uses play as a tool to explore issues around loss and grief and to correct any misconceptions.

P3 A variety of materials and approaches are used to facilitate the expression and resolution of issues related to bereavement.

SUB TOPIC Cont.   **SUPPORT FOR GRIEF AND BEREAVEMENT ISSUES**

PROCESSES
: P4 The play specialist discusses the goals of play interventions and ongoing observations with parents/carers.

: P5 The play specialist ensures that the issues identified are documented and shared with the key professionals in the child's life

OUTCOMES
: O1 Play interventions to address bereavement issues for identified children are planned, implemented and evaluated.

: O2 All the relevant professionals in the child's life are kept informed.

SUB TOPIC   **SAFEGUARDING CHILDREN**

CARE GROUP
: Children aged 2 years and over

STANDARD

OBJECTIVE
: To ensure that children are able to communicate anything that is causing them anxiety through play. These anxieties will be responded to appropriately.

: Observations of children at play contribute to diagnosis. Care plans for vulnerable children include play.

RATIONALE
: Children's play and creative work reflects their internal and external life experiences and provides valuable insights into their anxieties. A percentage of children admitted to hospital will have experienced abuse in some form and they may reveal this, consciously or unconsciously, in their play. Play specialists observe and assess all children at play and their interactions with family members. This routine screening of themes and behaviours is unobtrusive and can contribute to the identification of children at risk.

: Children who are failing to thrive may respond positively to the stimulation and enjoyment of hospital play activities. Observation of these play activities can contribute to the assessment process and care plan.

STRUCTURES
: S1 Play specialists attend training on child protection and local procedures. They attend regular child protection updates.

: S2 The contribution of play specialists to child protection is recognised. Play specialists attend multi-professional meetings and have access to expert advice and extended study opportunities.

: S3 Play specialists ensure all volunteer and student workers on placement have enhanced CRB clearance.

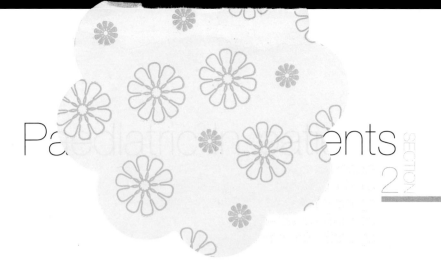

PAEDIATRIC IN-PATIENTS

SUB TOPIC Cont. | **SAFEGUARDING CHILDREN**

STRUCTURES

S4 Volunteer and student workers are given clear guidelines on local procedures for safe guarding children.

S5 Volunteer and student workers wear identification.

S6 Play specialists have access to clinical supervision and counselling when engaged in child protection work.

PROCESSES

P1 Observations of children at play, on their own, with other children or with family members provide opportunities for play specialists to screen for unusual interactions, themes and behaviours.

P2 Referrals for formal assessments of developmental abilities and verbal and non-verbal interactions with family members in cases where there are child protection concerns are processed and dealt with by the play team.

P3 Planned play programmes to support children who have experienced neglect or abuse are implemented as part of the care plan.

P4 The play specialist uses play and the relationship developed through it, to support anxious, distressed and disturbed children where there are child protection concerns.

P5 The play specialist undertakes preparation for physical examination in child abuse investigations respecting the additional psychological vulnerability of these children.

P6 The play specialist recognises professional boundaries in child abuse cases.

OUTCOMES

O1 Children's verbalised or played out communications are responded to appropriately.

O2 Disclosures of abuse and observations that suggest abuse are treated confidentially. Local policies for reporting are followed.

O3 Accurate contemporaneous written records are completed to support child protection work.

O4 Drawings or writing produced by children are dated, timed and signed and stored in the child's notes.

O5 Social work and police investigations are supported in cases of alleged abuse.

PAEDIATRIC IN-PATIENTS

SUB TOPIC   **SIBLING SUPPORT**

CARE GROUP   The siblings of children aged 2 to 12 years

STANDARD

OBJECTIVE   To provide support for the siblings of in-patient children.

RATIONALE   Recognising and meeting the needs of siblings who visit the hospital is one way in which play specialists deliver family centred care. Healthy siblings need play activities to help them settle on the ward and to ensure that their playful energy has a safe outlet. Siblings may be distressed or anxious about the hospitalisation of their brother or sister and the resulting disruption to family life. Play specialists acknowledge their feelings through play and conversation.

STRUCTURES   S1 Staffing levels allow for the safe supervision of siblings in the playroom.

S2 Sufficient space and equipment is available enabling siblings to join in with playroom activities.

S3 Sibling support is recognised as a valuable part of family centred care and is included in play specialist job descriptions and work plans.

PROCESSES   P1 The play specialist gathers information about siblings from parents/carers. This will include sibling responses to the hospital admission. The play specialist offers support and advice where necessary.

P2 The play specialist observes sibling play and interactions for signs of disturbance and misconceptions. The play specialist responds directly or indirectly to allow the expression of concerns and offer support.

P3 The play specialist helps sibling to understand what is happening to their ill brother or sister. The play specialist enables siblings to explore with their feelings when a sibling has suffered a major trauma or is terminally ill.

OUTCOMES   O1 Siblings who visit the ward are able to engage in play activities.

O2 Play specialist observations of siblings contribute to family centred care.

O3 Where additional work has been undertaken with siblings, there is liaison with the key professionals in the child's life.

O4 Siblings who visit the ward have access to a range of enjoyable play activities.

YOUNG PEOPLE

SUB TOPIC   **CREATION AND MAINTENANCE OF AN AGE APPROPRIATE ENVIRONMENT**

CARE GROUP   All patients using designated adolescent spaces

STANDARD

OBJECTIVE   To create and maintain a welcoming environment for young people where social and recreational activities take place. Health and safety guidelines are followed

RATIONALE   Current Department of Health guidance5 recommends that young people are cared for in designated adolescent units. The provision of age appropriate décor and activities enhances the hospital experience for this age group. Play specialists are trained to involve young people in the creation and maintenance of an age appropriate environment.

STRUCTURES   S1 Space for social and recreational activities is adequate and within reach of medical and nursing staff.

S2 Play specialists who work in adolescent services attend training on adolescent issues.

S3 Funds are provided for appropriate and up-to-date recreational equipment and décor.

S4 Play specialists receive clear guidance and training on risk management procedures for the use of electrical equipment, theft, damage, child protection, internet access, drug and alcohol abuse, smoking and infection control.

S5 Ward managers, modern matrons and play specialists have mechanisms in place for liaison regarding the adolescent environment, equipment and film media.

S6 Sufficient funding is allocated to allow the periodic review and renewal of recreational equipment.

S7 New play specialists, volunteers and students are provided with written information about infection control and risk management practices within each recreation or play area.

S9 The recreation environment is culturally inclusive. Games, books, music and equipment appropriate and sufficient to the age, developmental stage, gender, ethnicity and special needs of patients are provided.

PROCESSES   P1 Play specialists involve adolescent patients in the creation of appealing recreation areas and visual displays.

P2 Play specialists store equipment safely and ensure that the necessary cleaning takes place.

YOUNG PEOPLE

SUB TOPIC Cont.   **CREATION AND MAINTENANCE OF AN AGE APPROPRIATE ENVIRONMENT**

PROCESSES   P3 Play specialists provide recreational equipment that is suitable for adolescents and reflects a diversity of cultures.

P4 Play specialists monitor and advise staff, patients and their parents/carers on the viewing of legally permissible PC games and films.

P5 Play specialists maintain an awareness of new products and trends and involve users in planning for new purchases and any changes.

OUTCOMES   O1 Young people recognise areas that have been designed with their interests in mind.

O2 Young people use social or recreation areas which have been designated for their use.

O3 Young people demonstrate respect for the activities and equipment within any designated areas.

O4 Risks in designated areas are minimised.

SUB TOPIC   **PROVISION OF RECREATIONAL AND THERAPEUTIC ACTIVITIES**

CARE GROUP STANDARD   All patients using designated adolescent spaces

OBJECTIVE   Patients are provided with a range of activities to promote their social, cognitive and emotional development, encourage adaptation to the hospital environment and contribute to the achievement of medical and nursing objectives.

RATIONALE   The adolescent in hospital is emotionally vulnerable. The hospital environment, illness, and nursing interventions restrict normal behaviour. Recreational and therapeutic activities promote normal behaviour and provide an outlet for emotions.

STRUCTURES   S1 A play specialist is employed to provide and facilitate activities for adolescent patients.

S2 The adolescent activity programme receives sufficient core funding to ensure activities are up-to-date and appealing to young people.

S3 Suitable space is allocated for the provision of an activity programme for young people.

S4 Adolescent patients with restricted mobility or mental health issues are given equal access to activity programmes.

YOUNG PEOPLE

SUB TOPIC Cont. **PROVISION OF RECREATIONAL AND THERAPEUTIC ACTIVITIES**

STRUCTURES

S5 Regular meetings where all members of the multi disciplinary team are able to review and plan individual care for adolescents, take place.

S6 Care plans include recognition of the need for recreation and social interaction, and contributions from play specialists.

PROCESSES

P1 The play specialist promotes adaptation to the in-patient setting by welcoming new patients, assessing their interests, introducing the activity programme and talking about the role of the play specialist.

P2 The play specialist leads activities suitable for groups and encourages patient participation.

P3 The play specialist provides creative activities that promote self expression.

P4 Activities to promote self-esteem, positive body image, social interaction and peer support are provided.

P5 The play specialist liaises with members of the multi-disciplinary team to support the implementation of care plans.

P6 Young people are provided with activities that enable them to experience success and see that their endeavours are valued.

P7 The play specialist documents patient names, ages and the type of play services accessed for clinical governance purposes.

OUTCOMES

O1 Young people are able to participate in a range of activities reducing the risk of negative experiences whilst in hospital.

O2 Young people in hospital feel that their individual needs, interests and concerns have been understood and responded to.

O3 Young people in hospital are able to access the play service regularly.

O4 Play service numerical data is collated and published periodically.

YOUNG PEOPLE

SUB TOPIC   **PROVISION OF PRE-ADMISSION INFORMATION AND SUPPORT**

CARE GROUP   Patients aged 13 to their nineteenth birthday and their families due to be admitted to the hospital

STANDARD   STANDARD

OBJECTIVE   To provide meaningful and accessible information to young people and their families prior to admission. To provide physical and psychological preparation

RATIONALE   Adolescents should be provided with clear, age appropriate information, in order to dispel any misconceptions they may have. Information material should address the concerns of young people. Concerns around privacy, consent, independence and peer support during hospital admissions are common in this age group.

STRUCTURES
- S1 Age appropriate information provision is part of the clinical governance requirements of the ward or unit.
- S2 Play specialists are aware of the processes for consultation, advice and approval of written information for patients and their families.
- S3 Internet pages, booklets, videos, photographs or information sheets are produced specifically for young people and their families.
- S4 Funding and equipment for developing information material is available to play specialists.
- S5 Play specialists are able to allocate time to the development of information material.
- S6 Mechanisms exist for the translation of information material into languages reflecting the ethnicity of the local population.

PROCESSES
- P1 Information written by play specialists for patients is reviewed and approved by members of staff working with young people prior to use.
- P2 The source of all information used is clearly identified and dated.
- P3 The most effective means of delivering appropriate information are identified through training, consultation and research.
- P4 Young people and their families are consulted as part of the development process.
- P5 Audits are undertaken to analyse patient uptake of information.

OUTCOMES
- O1 Patients and their families receive timely, meaningful information prior to admission to hospital.
- O2 Patients and their families are able to seek further support and information if they so wish.

YOUNG PEOPLE

SUB TOPIC   **PREPARATION FOR INVESTIGATIONS, SURGERY AND MEDICAL PROCEDURES**

CARE GROUP   All patients using designated adolescent spaces

STANDARD

OBJECTIVE   Patients are able to understand, at a developmentally appropriate level, the procedure they are to experience. To enable patients to develop adaptive coping strategies. To enable patients to participate in the consent process.

RATIONALE   The UN Convention on the Rights of the Child states that the child has the right to be fully involved in decisions about his care. In order to reduce misconceptions and anxieties and enable participation in the consent process, young people need appropriate preparation and education. Preparation can aid effective pain management.

STRUCTURES   S1 Play specialist hours of employment enable them to assess, plan and implement preparation programmes when required.

S2 Adolescent units have mechanisms in place to ensure play specialists are informed of planned procedures.

S3 Play specialists undertake ongoing education to ensure excellence in preparation techniques for this age group. This includes reflective practice, peer review, professional conferences and local teaching sessions.

PROCESSES   P1 The play specialist gathers information about the young person requiring preparation through observation and interaction with the young person and dialogue with family and staff members.

P2 Parents/carers have the reasons for preparation and the approach to be taken explained to them.

P3 The play specialist selects the most appropriate method and materials for the preparation session after carrying out an assessment of the young person.

P4 The play specialist explains the forthcoming procedure using a variety of suitable visual media, monitoring verbal and non-verbal communication throughout, in one or more sessions.

P5 The play specialist halts preparation if the young person shows undue anxiety or wishes to cease the session. The play specialist explores the possible reasons for this anxiety at an appropriate time.

P6 The play specialist acknowledges anxiety about pain and works collaboratively with staff and parents/carers to address concerns.

YOUNG PEOPLE

SUB TOPIC Cont.   **PREPARATION FOR INVESTIGATIONS, SURGERY AND MEDICAL PROCEDURES**

PROCESSES   P7 The play specialist informs parents/carers of the outcome of the preparation and coping strategies identified.

P8 The play specialist reports directly to the nurse caring for the young person and documents the content and outcome of preparation in patient's notes.

OUTCOMES   O1 Young people comprehend, as fully as they wish to, the details of medical and surgical procedures.

O2 Parents/carers are informed of the purpose, content and outcome of preparation.

O3 The record of preparation is accessible to all health professionals involved in the young person's care.

SUB TOPIC   **POST-TREATMENT OR POST-PROCEDURAL SUPPORT**

CARE GROUP   Patients aged 13 years to their nineteenth birthday who have undergone surgery or an invasive procedure

STANDARD

OBJECTIVE   Play specialists ensure that young people have the opportunity to reflect on and gain further information about their experience of invasive or investigative treatment or procedures. To enable young people to share concerns they may have.

RATIONALE   Experience of hospitalisation and illness, particularly when needles or invasive procedures have been involved can arouse anxiety in young people, which can impair their coping abilities. With support, young people can be helped to make sense of difficult experiences.

Debriefing conversations and/or creative activities can encourage self-expression and reflection.

STRUCTURES   S1 Play specialists allocate time to see patients following invasive medical and surgical procedures.

S2 Regular liaison with members of the multi-disciplinary team takes place allowing post procedural work to be planned, assessed and discussed.

S3 Opportunities for clinical supervision and reflective practice are provided for play specialists. Play specialists are enabled to develop knowledge and expertise in this area of work.

YOUNG PEOPLE

SUB TOPIC Cont.	**POST-TREATMENT OR POST-PROCEDURAL SUPPORT**

PROCESSES

P1 The play specialist gathers information about the young person's experiences during the procedure from the family and staff members involved.

P2 The play specialist facilitates therapeutic post-procedural conversation or activities acknowledging the patient's experiences and feelings.

P3 Positive coping techniques and helpful behaviours are identified and reinforced.

P4 The outcome of post-procedural work is shared with parents/carers. Advice and suggestions for ongoing support are given.

OUTCOMES

O1 Young people are helped to make sense of difficult experiences with support from play specialists.

O2 Parents/carers feel able to help their adolescent adjust to the hospital experience.

O3 There is effective communication around post-procedural care within the multi-disciplinary team. Patients with particular problems are referred on appropriately.

O4 The play specialist provides a report of post-procedural work in the patient's notes.

SUB TOPIC	**COPING SKILLS EDUCATION**

CARE GROUP

Patients aged 13 years to their nineteenth birthday having clinical investigations or treatment

STANDARD

OBJECTIVE

Play specialists assist young people to cope effectively with clinical procedures and investigations by enabling them to choose, rehearse and use techniques that help them to manage their feelings and responses.

RATIONALE

Coping skills; breathing techniques and alternative focus activities, can help a young person to cope during a procedure. The young person is therefore less likely to be distressed and non-compliant, which creates a safer clinical environment. The young person can gain confidence in themselves and those who care for them.

STRUCTURES

S1 Play specialists are informed of planned procedures. Referral pathways are in place for young people showing additional anxiety.

S2 Play specialists undertake ongoing education to ensure excellence in coping skills education.

YOUNG PEOPLE

SUB TOPIC Cont.   **COPING SKILLS EDUCATION**

PROCESSES

P1 The play specialist gathers information about the procedure. The play specialist establishes a plan in conjunction with the young person and the members of staff involved in the procedure.

P2 A range of coping skills are discussed with the young person and their benefits explained. One or two methods are chosen and, if time allows, rehearsed prior to the event.

P3 The play specialist works collaboratively with staff to ensure that the young person can make choices where possible and is involved in decisions around procedures to be carried out.

P4 If the play specialist is to be present to support the young person during the procedure; the role he/ she will take is described to the family and staff members involved.

P5 Where the play specialist is not accompanying the young person, the family and staff members involved are given clear information about the chosen coping skills.

P6 The play specialist praises specific achievements and positive coping behaviours.

P7 Coping behaviours and outcomes are documented in the patient's notes.

OUTCOMES

O1 Young people are provided with knowledge and skills to help reduce their anxiety during procedures.

O2 Parents/carers understand the purpose and support the process of coping skills education.

O3 A record of the coping skills strategies employed is accessible to all health professionals involved in the young person's care

SUB TOPIC   **THERAPEUTIC INTERVENTIONS**

CARE GROUP   Patients aged 13 years to their nineteenth birthday where there is an identified concern

STANDARD

OBJECTIVE   Issues which arise as a result of hospital experiences, illness or treatment are identified and responded to using a range of age appropriate therapeutic techniques.

RATIONALE   Illness and/or hospital experiences in adolescence may cause short or long term psychological harm. Raised anxiety levels have an impact on medical and nursing care. Young people who are identified as having increased anxieties can benefit from additional therapeutic support.

YOUNG PEOPLE

SUB TOPIC Cont.   **THERAPEUTIC INTERVENTIONS**

STRUCTURES

S1 The play specialist team includes staff with considerable experience who can lead and guide therapeutic interventions.

S2 The play specialist team work schedule is organised to allow time for one-to-one therapeutic work.

S3 Play specialists have regular contact with members of the psychology team for clinical supervision for therapeutic work.

S4 Play specialists attend regular multi-professional team meetings where therapeutic work can be discussed and patients referred on if required.

S5 Structures exist to ensure information about atypical behaviour is shared.

PROCESSES

P1 Play specialists observe and assess young people's verbal and non-verbal communication during recreational and social interactions for atypical behaviour or patterns.

P2 Play specialists take referrals from team members to address specific concerns, for example anxiety about needles.

P3 Therapeutic interventions are planned, implemented and evaluated during one or more in-patient admissions or on an out-patient basis.

P4 A variety of materials and approaches are used to initiate mastery of anxieties, reflection on and the resolution of issues related to the hospital experience or treatment.

P5 Play specialists discuss the goals of therapeutic interventions and ongoing observations with parents/carers.

OUTCOMES

O1 Parents/carers are kept informed about therapeutic interventions.

O2 Young people identified by the play specialist, parents or members of the multi-disciplinary team, as having increased anxieties are provided with additional support through planned therapeutic interventions.

O3 All the relevant professionals are informed of the content and outcomes of the interventions.

O4 Plans, content and outcomes of therapeutic interventions are recorded in the patient's notes.

YOUNG PEOPLE

SUB TOPIC   **ISOLATION**

CARE GROUP
: Young people who require isolation due to reduced immunity, infectious conditions or radioactivity.

STANDARD

OBJECTIVE
: To provide activity programmes for young people who require isolation. To provide sensory stimulation. To address misconceptions or anxieties.

RATIONALE
: Young people in isolation are cut off from social interaction and the support of friends. Formal and informal activity programmes developed by play specialists provide regular opportunities for social and recreational activities and an outlet for feelings.

STRUCTURES
: S1 There are sufficient play specialists to run activity programmes for young people in isolation.

: S2 The activity programme funding is sufficient to provide for the additional resources required by isolation patients.

: S3 Structures and mechanisms exist to ensure that all members of the multi-disciplinary team communicate about isolation patients.

PROCESSES
: P1 Play specialists provide a wide range of stimulating recreational activities.

: P2 Play specialists provide activities to address the restricted social environment and maintain links with the outside world.

: P3 Play specialists support parents/carers and staff to lead activities in the isolation environment.

: P4 Play specialists ensure that the cleaning, disposal and storage of equipment for isolation patients is undertaken following established health and safety and infection control guidelines.

: P5 Play specialists acknowledge the emotional difficulties associated with isolation for young people through active listening and supportive conversation.

OUTCOMES
: O1 Patients in isolation receive regular, planned input from play specialists. This is geared to their individual needs.

: O2 The developmental and psychological risks associated with isolating young people are reduced through the implementation of activity programmes.

: O3 Health and safety policies are adhered to.

YOUNG PEOPLE

SUB TOPIC **SAFEGUARDING YOUNG PEOPLE**

CARE GROUP   All in patients aged 17 years and under

STANDARD

OBJECTIVE   To ensure that the anxieties of young people in hospital are responded to appropriately. To ensure observations of young people during recreational activities contribute to diagnosis. To ensure that recreational and therapeutic activity is part of the care plan for vulnerable young people.

RATIONALE   Young people's creative work, social and recreational activities reflect their internal and external life experiences and provide valuable insights into their anxieties. A percentage of young people admitted to hospital will have experienced abuse. They may reveal this consciously or unconsciously during activities. A young person may choose to disclose information about abusive or anxiety producing experiences to the play specialist as a result of the relationship developed.

Where abuse has been identified, social activities and the relationship with the play specialist can contribute to the support given to a vulnerable young person.

STRUCTURES   S1 Play specialists attend training on child protection, local procedures, and regular child protection updates.

S2 The contribution of play specialists to child protection is recognised. Play specialists attend multi-professional meetings and have access to expert advice and extended study opportunities.

S3 All volunteer and student workers on placement have enhanced CRB clearance.

S4 Volunteer and student workers are given clear guidelines on local procedures for safe guarding young people.

S5 Volunteer and student workers wear identification.

S6 Play specialists have access to clinical supervision and counselling when engaged in child protection work.

PROCESSES   P1 Play specialists screen for unusual interactions, themes and behaviours, when observing young people engaged in solitary or social activities with peers or family members.

P2 Formal assessments of developmental abilities and verbal and non-verbal interactions with family members are undertaken by play specialists in cases where there are child protection concerns.

YOUNG PEOPLE

SUB TOPIC Cont.   **SAFEGUARDING YOUNG PEOPLE**

PROCESSES   P3 Planned activity programmes are implemented as part of the care plan.

P4 Play specialists use activities and the relationship developed through them, to support anxious, distressed and disturbed young people where there are child protection concerns.

P5 Play specialists take a proactive approach to maintaining professional boundaries by explaining the scope of their role and restricting social activity to that required for professional purposes. Patients are referred to the psychosocial support services where necessary.

OUTCOMES   O1 Young people's verbalised or acted out communications are heard and responded to appropriately.

O2 Disclosures of abuse and observations that suggest abuse are treated confidentiality. Local policies for reporting observations are followed.

O3 Accurate, contemporaneous written records are completed to support child protection work.

O4 Risk taking behaviours are noted and discussed.

O5 Any drawings, writing or other materials produced by a young person where there is a concern of abuse, are stored in the notes, dated, timed and signed by the play specialist.

O6 Social work and police investigations are supported in cases of alleged abuse.

SUB TOPIC   **TRANSITION**

CARE GROUP   Patients moving from paediatric and adolescent services to adult health services

STANDARD

OBJECTIVE   Patients are assisted in making a purposeful and planned transition from adolescent to adult services.

RATIONALE   The transfer to adult services can be abrupt and disorientating for young people and their families. As a result, some patients are lost to medical supervision altogether at this time. An increasing number of chronically ill children are surviving into adulthood. Both the patients and health service providers value a seamless transfer facilitated by the multi-disciplinary team.

YOUNG PEOPLE

SUB TOPIC Cont.   **TRANSITION**

STRUCTURES   S1 Paediatric and adolescent units have structures and policies in place to guide the transition process.

S2 Play specialists establish networks with their colleagues in other specialties.

S3 Play specialists receive training and support to guide their work in transition.

S4 Mechanisms exist to ensure play specialists are informed about young people who are moving to adult services.

PROCESSES   P1 Play specialists participate in the multi-disciplinary team approach to the planning and implementation of the transition processes for patients.

P2 Play specialists contribute to multi-disciplinary transition planning documentation.

P3 Play specialists take an active role in preparing patients for the transition to adult services.

P4 Play specialists use a variety of materials and approaches to support transition education. Transition education includes preparation for the emotional responses to change.

OUTCOMES   O1 Patients transferring to adult health services receive support and guidance from play specialists.

O2 Documentation on transition to adult services is maintained.

BABIES AND INFANTS

SUB TOPIC   **CREATION AND MAINTENANCE OF AN AGE APPROPRIATE ENVIRONMENT**

CARE GROUP   Patients aged two years old and under

STANDARD

OBJECTIVE   Parents/carers of babies and infants are able to access play facilities and obtain clean, stimulating toys and play equipment.

RATIONALE   Play is a basic requirement for normal health and development. Without the provision of supervised play environments, play opportunities for babies can be limited and normal development restricted. Lack of structured and supervised play can lead to an increase in adverse incidents.

STRUCTURES   S1 Playrooms/areas cater for babies and infants. There is safe floor space for crawling, first steps and toddling.

S2 The size and layout of the play environment is sufficient for parents/carers and staff to accompany babies and participate in play.

S3 There is ample storage for play equipment, which is cleaned regularly.

S4 Play specialists receive training and guidance on risk management, which includes infection control, the use of electrical equipment, theft, damage and manual handling.

S5 The special requirements of babies and infants with restricted mobility and/or special needs are taken into account when funding and designing play environments.

S6 Ward managers, modern matrons and play specialists have mechanisms in place for liaison out play environments.

S7 Sufficient funding is allocated to allow the periodic review and renewal of play equipment.

S8 New play specialists, volunteers and students are provided with written information about risk management procedures for each play environment.

S9 The play environment provided for babies and infants is culturally inclusive. Play materials, books, music and equipment appropriate and sufficient to the age, developmental stage, gender, ethnicity and special needs of patients are provided.

PROCESSES   P1 Toys and games are stored away to enable the cleaning of the playroom to take place.

P2 Play specialists organise and set out a range of play activities after assessing patient needs. The seasonal and religious calendar and staffing ratios are also taken into account.

BABIES AND INFANTS

SUB TOPIC Cont. **CREATION AND MAINTENANCE OF AN AGE APPROPRIATE ENVIRONMENT**

PROCESSES

P3 Play specialists maintain their awareness of new play products and involve parents and staff in planning for new purchases and any changes.

P4 Play specialists provide toys and equipment that is suitable for babies and infants.

P5 Play specialists encourage parents/carers to use play equipment, and give advice about appropriate play activities. Parents/carers are directed to toy cupboards.

P6 Play specialists ensure that the regular washing of toys and equipment used by babies takes place in accordance with local infection control policies.

P7 Play specialists advise parents/carers and staff on what to do when a baby has finished with a toy that requires washing.

OUTCOMES

O1 Babies and infants are able to engage in play activities daily, in a safe and clean environment.

O2 Parents/carers and staff enter the play environment and demonstrate respect for the activities and equipment.

O3 Parents/carers and staff are encouraged and able to use a range of age appropriate toys.

O4 Risks in designated play areas are minimised.

SUB TOPIC **ACTIVITIES TO PROMOTE NORMAL GROWTH AND DEVELOPMENT**

CARE GROUP Patients who have reached full term at 2 years of age

STANDARD

OBJECTIVE To ensure that developmental progress is maintained during a hospital admission.

RATIONALE Normal development is at risk from delay and/or damage from lengthy or repeated hospital admissions. Babies or infants who are nursed in isolation are at risk from sensory deprivation. The provision of appropriate stimulation, play and communication reduces these risks.

STRUCTURES

S1 The play specialist team includes staff with the appropriate knowledge and skills to lead and guide developmental play programmes for babies.

S2 The requirements for developmentally stimulating play for babies who have a range of abilities are considered when purchasing equipment and setting budgets.

BABIES AND INFANTS

SUB TOPIC Cont.   **ACTIVITIES TO PROMOTE NORMAL GROWTH AND DEVELOPMENT**

STRUCTURES   S3 Play specialists meet with members of the multi-disciplinary team (physiotherapists, speech and language therapists, dieticians and occupational therapists) to discuss the developmental needs of patients.

S4 Play specialists contribute to the shared documentation of the developmental goals for each patient.

S5 Play specialists receive training in the infection control procedures and health and safety requirements that relate directly to their work with babies and infants.

PROCESSES   P1 Play specialists assess the developmental needs and progress of babies who have repeat admissions or who are hospitalised for long periods, and document their observations.

P2 Developmental assessments are included in structured play programmes for babies who are hospitalised for several days.

P3 Babies are provided with a range of appealing sensory experiences and interesting activities.

P4 Play specialists adapt play activities to suit patients who have restricted movement and/or special needs.

P5 Play specialists provide guidance for parents/carers on how to play with their babies taking into account the restrictions created by medical equipment.

OUTCOMES   O1 The risk of developmental delay due to hospitalisation is minimised by the provision of a wide range of enjoyable, developmentally stimulating play activities.

O2 Babies and infants have access to developmentally appropriate play activities.

O3 Parental bonding is facilitated in the hospital environment.

O4 Co-ordination between health professionals and parents ensures developmental health is optimised.

BABIES AND INFANTS

SUB TOPIC	**MAINTAINING LINKS WITH HOME AND FAMILIAR ROUTINES**
CARE GROUP	Patients aged two years and under especially those who have an extended stay in hospital
STANDARD	
OBJECTIVE	Play specialists demonstrate an awareness of familiar routines and behaviours in their communication and care. Babies are enabled to retain an awareness of their home life and their place in it, through the play activities provided by the play specialist. The integrity of family life is respected, cultural differences acknowledged and the development of domestic language encouraged.
RATIONALE	Hospitalisation involves a separation from much that is familiar and predictable. It is important that babies and infants are enabled to make the transition home after an admission with minimal anxiety. By leading domestic play incorporating culturally familiar activities and using images and sounds from home, play specialists actively keep family life to the fore. For babies who have spent their lives in hospital, the introduction to domestic activity through play is vital.
STRUCTURES	S1 Care plans include recognition of the need to maintain familiar routines, and contributions from play specialists.
	S2 Play specialists are able to allocate sufficient time to this aspect of care.
	S3 Play specialists promote an awareness of separation anxiety within the multi-disciplinary team.
	S4 Play specialists attend training on diversity and spirituality.
PROCESSES	P1 Play specialists use a variety of play activities to stimulate sensory pathways, enabling the baby to retain an awareness of family, friends and the home environment.
	P2 Play specialists acknowledge the significance of the baby's belongings, preferences and routines through play activities and dialogue with parents/carers.
	P3 Play specialists enquire about and have respect for family routines and preferences.
	P4 Play specialists involve parents/carers in play activities, maintaining links with home and family.
	P5 Play specialists engage pre-verbal babies in play about home life and people.

BABIES AND INFANTS

SUB TOPIC Cont.   **MAINTAINING LINKS WITH HOME AND FAMILIAR ROUTINES**

PROCESSES   P6 For babies who have been in hospital since birth or for long periods of time, details and images of milestones, achievements and significant hospital staff are recorded in a "memory book" for the baby to take home on discharge.

P7 Play specialists introduce play activities which prepare for child for discharge home.

OUTCOMES   O1 Maladaptive behaviours associated with separation from home, family and predictable routines are minimised.

O2 Baby retains his identity as a member of the family.

O3 Parental anxiety before and after discharge is minimised.

O4 Developmental progress is sustained through the use of domestic play and conversation.

SUB TOPIC   **THERAPEUTIC PLAY ACTIVITIES**

CARE GROUP   Patients aged two years and under

STANDARD

OBJECTIVE   Issues which arise as a result of hospital experiences, illness or treatment are identified and responded to using a range of therapeutic techniques.

RATIONALE   Illness and/or hospital experiences in childhood may cause short or long term psychological harm. Babies and infants can suffer from sensory deprivation or disorientation, food aversion and/or increased anxiety. Babies or infants who are identified as suffering from increased anxiety are provided with additional support through therapeutic play sessions.

STRUCTURES   S1 The play specialist team includes staff with considerable experience who can support and guide therapeutic interventions with babies and infants.

S2 The play specialist work schedule is organised to permit flexibility for one-to-one work.

S3 Play specialists attend regular multi-professional team meetings where developmental and therapeutic work is discussed and patients referred on if required.

PROCESSES   P1 The play specialist observes and assesses infant behaviour during medical interventions and interactions with parents/carers to identify patterns or atypical responses.

BABIES AND INFANTS

SUB TOPIC Cont.	**THERAPEUTIC PLAY ACTIVITIES**
PROCESSES	P2 Therapeutic interventions are planned, implemented and evaluated in conjunction with members of the multi-disciplinary team.
	P3 The play specialist uses a variety of methods and approaches to resolve identified issues, using his/her knowledge of the sensory and emotional needs of babies.
	P4 The play specialist discusses the goals of therapeutic interventions and ongoing observations with parents/carers and staff.
	P5 The play specialist ensures that the issues identified are documented and shared with the key professionals in the baby's life.
OUTCOMES	O1 Planned additional interventions are provided for babies where specific concerns have been identified.
	O2 Parents/carers are informed about therapeutic activities.
	O3 All the relevant professionals in the patient's life are involved and informed.
	O4 Play specialist interventions to address specific concerns support medical and nursing care.

SUB TOPIC	**SAFEGUARDING CHILDREN**
CARE GROUP	Patients aged two years and under
STANDARD	STANDARD
OBJECTIVE	To ensure that staff members observe and assess behaviours and interactions with family members To ensure that established policies are adhered to.
RATIONALE	Playtime provides an opportunity for observation. Young children's play reflects their internal and external life experiences and provides valuable insights into anxieties and the nature of relationships with family members. A percentage of children admitted to hospital have experienced abuse. They may reveal this consciously or unconsciously through play.
	Babies and infants who are failing to thrive sometimes respond in an atypical manner to hospital play activities. Observations of play sessions contribute to diagnosis and care planning.

BABIES AND INFANTS

SUB TOPIC Cont.   **SAFEGUARDING CHILDREN**

STRUCTURES

S1 Play specialists attend training on child protection, local procedures, and regular updates.

S2 The contribution of play specialists to child protection is recognised. Play specialists attend multi-professional meetings and have access to expert advice and extended study opportunities.

S3 Play specialists ensure all volunteer and student workers on placement have enhanced CRB clearance.

S4 Volunteer and student workers are given clear guidelines on local procedures for safe guarding children.

S5 Volunteer and student workers wear identification.

S6 Play specialists have access to clinical supervision and counselling when engaged in child protection work.

PROCESSES

P1 Play specialists screen for unusual interactions, themes and behaviours, when observing babies and infants engaged in solitary or social play or with family members.

P2 Formal assessments of developmental abilities and verbal and non-verbal interactions with family members are undertaken by play specialists in cases where there are child protection concerns.

P3 Play programmes are included in care plans.

P4 Play specialists use play and the relationship developed through it, to support anxious, and/or distressed babies and infants where there are child protection concerns.

P5 Play specialists recognise their professional boundaries in child abuse cases.

OUTCOMES

O1 Atypical behaviours and played out communications are responded to appropriately.

O2 Disclosures of abuse and observations which suggest abuse are treated confidentially. Local policies for reporting observations are followed.

O3 Accurate, contemporaneous written records are completed to support child protection work.

O4 Social work and police investigations are supported in cases of alleged abuse.

BABIES AND INFANTS

SUB TOPIC	**SIBLING SUPPORT**
CARE GROUP	Siblings of patients aged two years and under
STANDARD	STANDARD
OBJECTIVE	To provide support for siblings.
RATIONALE	Recognising and meeting the needs of siblings who visit the hospital is one way in which play specialists deliver family centred care. Healthy siblings need play activities to help them settle on the ward and to ensure that their playful energy has a safe outlet. Siblings may be distressed by the hospitalisation of their baby brother or sister and the resulting disruption to family life. Play specialists acknowledge their feelings through play and conversation.

STRUCTURES

S1 Staffing levels allow for the safe supervision of siblings where appropriate.

S2 Sufficient space and equipment to allow siblings to engage in play activities is provided.

S3 Sibling support is included in play specialist job descriptions and work plans.

PROCESSES

P1 The play specialist gathers information about siblings from parents/carers. This will include sibling responses to the hospital admission. The play specialist offers support and advice where necessary.

P2 The play specialist welcomes sibling visitors to the ward and provides them with play activities.

P3 The play specialist observes sibling play and interactions, looking for signs of disturbance and misconceptions. The play specialist responds directly or indirectly to these. The play specialist offers support to the sibling.

P4 The play specialist addresses the needs of siblings to understand what is happening. The play specialist enables siblings to cope with their feelings where a sibling has suffered a major trauma or is terminally ill.

OUTCOMES

O1 Visiting siblings are able to engage in play activities.

O2 Play specialist observations of siblings contribute to family centred care.

O3 Where additional sibling work has been undertaken, liaison with key professionals in the child's life takes place.

O4 The hospital experiences of siblings include a range of enjoyable play activities.

BABIES AND INFANTS

SUB TOPIC   **MOVING FROM ONE CLINICAL SETTING TO ANOTHER**

CARE GROUP   Patients aged two years and under who have been in hospital for an extended period.

STANDARD

OBJECTIVE   To provide appropriate support for babies, infants and their primary carers when they are transferred from one clinical setting to another or discharged home. To provide preparation for the emotional and practical impacts of change.

RATIONALE   Visits to new wards, discussions about the practical arrangements and acknowledgment of the feelings associated with leaving a secure familiar environment will help parents/carers to feel less anxious. When babies are discharged home after an extended admission, parents/carers may be anxious about managing outside the supportive environment of the hospital. The play specialist is well placed to contribute to the planning process.

STRUCTURES   S1 The orientation programme for new play specialists includes meetings with staff on the wards to which babies may be transferred, health visitors and community professionals.

S2 Professional networks between play specialists across wards are maintained through joint meetings, training and shared projects.

S3 Staffing levels allow for play specialists to develop a range of materials to support transition processes.

PROCESSES   P1 Play specialists are informed when a baby is to move settings.

P2 Photographs of and written information about their destination are provided for parents/carers. Where possible, visits are arranged.

P3 Preparation information includes information about the staff on the new unit and the care provided there.

P4 The Information provided is adapted to recognise the emotional and physical state of the patient and family.

P5 Play specialists facilitate domestic play, discussions about home and "closure" activities with infants prior to discharge.

P6 Play specialists work with team members to ensure parents/ carers receive appropriate preparation for the emotional and practical implications of the transfer home.

BABIES AND INFANTS

SUB TOPIC Cont.   **MOVING FROM ONE CLINICAL SETTING TO ANOTHER**

OUTCOMES

O1 Infants being transferred from the ward are provided with sufficient age appropriate information about their destination and the staff they will meet there.

O2 Relevant practical information for parents/carers is provided prior to the transfer from the ward.

O3 Parents/carers' anxieties are acknowledged and managed through discussion and the provision of accurate information.

O4 Staff on receiving wards or in the community are given information about play activities for the child and developmental assessments undertaken on the ward.

OUT-PATIENT SETTINGS

SUB TOPIC   **CREATION AND MAINTENANCE OF AN AGE APPROPRIATE ENVIRONMENT**

CARE GROUP   Children in out-patient settings including the dependants of adult patients

STANDARD   STANDARD

OBJECTIVE   To create and maintain an environment where children of all developmental abilities visiting the out-patient department can play safely.

RATIONALE   Play is an essential part of childhood. It is an activity that can reduce tension. The provision of suitable play equipment in an out-patient department gives a clear message to children and their families that they are welcome and that the service is designed for them. It also encourages children to remain in one place thereby reducing potential conflicts with adult patients, traffic flow problems and the likelihood of unsafe play activity.

STRUCTURES   S1 There is consultation between clinic managers and play specialists over purchases of play equipment.

S2 Cleaning and storage arrangements are in line with infection control and risk management policies.

S3 Play specialists receive training and guidance on infection control and risk management procedures.

S4 A named person is responsible for the regular cleaning and inspection of play equipment.

PROCESSES   P1 Play equipment is regularly inspected for damage or faults, removed or replaced if necessary.

P2 Play facilities that maintain interest during an average waiting time and that are appropriate for children of all developmental abilities are provided.

P3 Where play facilities are unsupervised; parents/carers are notified of their responsibility to supervise their children.

OUTCOMES   O1 Children and their families feel welcome in the out-patient department and use the play facilities provided.

O2 Play equipment does not deteriorate or date, but is well maintained and renewed regularly.

O3 Cleaning and maintenance activity is recorded.

O4 Users are involved in the design and ongoing development of the service.

OUT-PATIENT SETTINGS

SUB TOPIC   **PROVISION OF RECREATIONAL AND THERAPEUTIC ACTIVITIES**

CARE GROUP   Children in out-patient settings including the dependants of adult patients

STANDARD

OBJECTIVE   Children are provided with a range of play activities under the supervision of a play specialist. Familiar toys, activities and staff members provide continuity for regular attendees.

RATIONALE   A visit to the hospital out-patient department may cause anxiety. The provision of play activities ensures that children feel welcome. It also provides opportunities for children to communicate their feelings and encourages the safe use of the space and equipment. Play specialist observations of children at play contribute to the assessment of the emotional state of attendees.

STRUCTURES   S1 Play specialists are employed to provide play activities in dedicated paediatric clinics.

S2 Sufficient storage space is allocated for the safe storage of play equipment.

S3 Sufficient funds are provided to purchase safe, appropriate toys, games, craft materials and large play equipment.

S4 Play specialists understand and adhere to local policies for the recruitment and supervision of volunteers.

S5 Play specialists meet regularly with clinic managers to discuss organisational issues.

S6 Suitable facilities for washing toys are provided close to the clinic and storage area.

S7 Play specialists receive training in the clinical specialities seen in the clinics.

S8 Play specialists are able to discuss concerns about physical or psychological issues that arise through interactions with children in the clinics with medical and nursing staff.

PROCESSES   P1 The play specialist plans activities according to the age range of attendees, clinic routines and the degree of intervention required.

P2 The space available for play is maximised without affecting the smooth running of the clinic or patient safety.

P3 Health education issues, cultural and religious festivals are reflected in the play activities provided.

P4 The play specialist undertakes formal assessments of developmental abilities of patients when requested by the clinic team.

OUT-PATIENT SETTINGS

SUB TOPIC Cont.   **PROVISION OF RECREATIONAL AND THERAPEUTIC ACTIVITIES**

PROCESSES

P5 The play specialist observes children at play, noting themes, physical abilities and interactions with real and/or imaginary people.

P6 Parents/carers are encouraged to join in with play activities and are informed of play specialist assessments and plans.

P7 The play specialist welcomes regular child attendees and recognises their need for continuity by providing familiar activities.

P8 The play specialist documents the names and ages of attendees and collates numerical data relating to the numbers of children using the play service on a daily basis.

OUTCOMES

O1 Children attending the out-patient department are able to participate, as fully as they wish or are able, in a range of play activities.

O2 Parents/carers have access to suitable play equipment.

O3 Observations which may contribute to the child's diagnosis and care are documented and verbally reported to the clinician.

O4 Play service numerical data is collated and published regularly. This is reported to the clinical governance committee.

SUB TOPIC   **INFORMATION ABOUT THE OUT-PATIENT SERVICE**

CARE GROUP

Patients and their families who have an appointment for an out-patient clinic

STANDARD

OBJECTIVE

To provide accessible and meaningful information to children and their families prior to their first out-patient appointment.

RATIONALE

A visit to the out-patient department is often the first step on a journey which starts with investigations and may end in a hospital admission. The child and family are likely to be anxious about what is involved and what the future holds. The geography of the hospital, clinic routines, the personnel and investigative procedures may all be new to them. Accurate information will reduce anxiety about practical arrangements and increase attendance rates and patient satisfaction.

Information in a variety of formats designed for children and appropriate to their level of understanding is effective.

OUT-PATIENT SETTINGS

| SUB TOPIC Cont. | INFORMATION ABOUT THE OUT-PATIENT SERVICE |

STRUCTURES

S1 Information provision is part of the clinical governance requirements for the out-patient service.

S2 Play specialists are aware of the processes for consultation, advice and approval of written information for patients and their families.

S3 Funding and equipment resources are available to play specialists developing information material.

S4 Mechanisms exist for the distribution of information to patients prior to their first clinic appointment.

S5 Audits are carried out to assess the effectiveness of the distribution and content of information.

S6 Mechanisms exist for the translation of information material into languages that reflect the ethnicity of the local population.

PROCESSES

P1 Play specialists develop information material for children.

P2 Visual material is used to add understanding.

P3 Children and their parents/carers are consulted when new information material for the out-patient services is being developed.

P4 Play specialists ensure all members of the clinic team are involved in the development of information material.

OUTCOMES

O1 Patients and their families receive meaningful information prior to an out-patient appointment.

O2 Patients and their families are able to seek further support and information if they so wish.

O3 Children arrive for their first clinic appointment prepared for the experience.

O4 The adults accompanying a child are aware of practical details; location of food outlets, play facilities, car parking arrangements and clinic routines.

O5 No child or family is excluded from receiving information because English is not their first language.

OUT-PATIENT SETTINGS

SUB TOPIC **PREPARATION FOR INVESTIGATIONS, SURGERY AND MEDICAL PROCEDURES**

CARE GROUP CARE GROUP Children and young people in the out patients department

STANDARD STANDARD

OBJECTIVE Patients are able to understand, at a developmentally appropriate level, the procedure they are to experience. To enable patients to develop adaptive coping strategies. To enable patients to participate in the consent process.

RATIONALE A child centred approach to preparation for procedures is needed.

Research has demonstrated that preparation through play reduces anxiety, supports effective pain management and encourages co-operative behaviour.

STRUCTURES S1 Play specialist hours of employment enable them to assess, plan and implement preparation programmes when required.

S2 Out-patient departments have mechanisms in place to ensure that play specialists are informed of planned procedures.

S3 Play specialists undertake ongoing education to ensure excellence in preparation techniques. This includes reflective practice, peer review, professional conferences and local teaching sessions.

PROCESSES P1 The play specialist gathers information about patient requiring preparation through observation and interaction with the child and dialogue with family and staff members.

P2 Parents/carers have the reasons for preparation and the approach to be taken explained to them.

P3 The play specialist selects the most appropriate method and materials for the preparation session after carrying out an assessment of the child.

P4 The play specialist engages the child in preparation play monitoring verbal and non- verbal communication throughout. For older children, t he play specialist explains the procedure and uses visual materials.

P5 The play specialist halts preparation play if the child shows undue anxiety. The possible reasons for anxiety are explored at an appropriate time.

P6 The play specialist acknowledges the child's anxiety about pain and works collaboratively with staff and carers to address this.

P7 Parents/carers are informed of the outcomes of the play preparation session. Coping strategies are identified.

OUT-PATIENT SETTINGS

SUB TOPIC Cont. **PREPARATION FOR INVESTIGATIONS, SURGERY AND MEDICAL PROCEDURES**

PROCESSES

P8 The play specialist reports directly to the child's nurse and documents the content and outcome of the preparation.

P9 Where possible, the play specialist returns to the child to facilitate post-procedural mastery play and debriefing.

OUTCOMES

O1 Age appropriate preparation for procedures, based on the circumstances of the individual child, is carried out in a timely fashion.

O2 Parents/carers are informed of the purpose, content and outcome of preparation.

O3 The record of preparation is accessible to all health professionals involved in the child's care.

SUB TOPIC **DISTRACTION THERAPY AND ALTERNATIVE FOCUS ACTIVITIES**

CARE GROUP Children having clinical procedures or investigations.

STANDARD STANDARD

OBJECTIVE To enable patients to cope effectively with clinical procedures and investigations by providing an alternative focus for their attention.

RATIONALE Distraction therapy and alternative focus activities help children to cope with procedures by diverting their attention. Children are less likely to be distressed and non-compliant, which creates a safer clinical environment. Children can gain confidence in themselves and those who care for them. As a result of the distraction therapy, the child may experience less pain.

STRUCTURES

S1 Play specialist hours of employment and staff ratios enable them to carry out distraction when required.

S2 Out-patient services have mechanisms in place to ensure that play specialists are informed of planned procedures.

S3 Play specialists undertake ongoing education to ensure excellence in distraction techniques.

S4 Funding for equipment for distraction is provided.

PROCESSES

P1 The play specialist gathers information about the child through observation, play and interaction.

P2 The play specialist gathers information about the procedure and establishes a plan in conjunction with the members of staff involved.

OUT-PATIENT SETTINGS

SUB TOPIC Cont. | **DISTRACTION THERAPY AND ALTERNATIVE FOCUS ACTIVITIES**

PROCESSES

P3 For older children, the distraction techniques to be used are discussed and rehearsed prior to the event.

P4 Distraction is carried out with respect for the safety of everyone involved. The roles of all staff members involved are respected.

P5 The play specialist praises specific achievements and positive coping behaviours and rewards with certificates and stickers, where appropriate.

P6 Distraction techniques and outcomes are documented in the child's notes.

OUTCOMES

O1 Age appropriate distraction therapy is carried out in a timely fashion.

O2 Parents/carers understand the purpose of and support the distraction.

O3 A record of distraction techniques is accessible to all health professionals involved in the child's care.

SUB TOPIC | **THERAPEUTIC PLAY ACTIVITIES**

CARE GROUP

Children and adolescents for whom there is a defined concern

STANDARD

OBJECTIVE

Issues which arise for children as a result of hospital experiences, illness or treatment are identified and responded to using a range of age appropriate therapeutic techniques.

RATIONALE

Illness and/or hospital experiences in childhood may cause short or long term psychological harm. Children and adolescents for whom there is a defined concern are provided with additional support through the provision of therapeutic play activities.

STRUCTURES

S1 The play specialist team includes staff with considerable experience who can lead and guide therapeutic work.

S2 The play specialist' work schedule is organised to permit flexibility for one-to-one therapeutic work on an out-patient basis.

S3 Play specialists receive regular clinical supervision for therapeutic work.

S4 Medical and nursing staff are aware of the additional therapeutic work carried out by play specialists and know how to refer patients to the play service.

S5 Play specialists attend regular multi-professional team meetings where therapeutic work is discussed and patients referred on if required.

S6 Play specialists participate in continuing education to maintain and develop their knowledge of therapeutic techniques.

Paediatric Out-patient Settings

OUT-PATIENT SETTINGS

SUB TOPIC Cont.   **THERAPEUTIC PLAY ACTIVITIES**

PROCESSES   P1 Therapeutic play interventions are planned, implemented and evaluated within one or more sessions on an out-patient basis.

P2 Liaison with nursing and medical staff ensures accurate information is gathered and joint planning can take place.

P3 A variety of materials and approaches are used to initiate mastery play and the exploration of anxieties and the resolution of issues related to the hospital experience, illness or an anticipated event.

P4 Control and choice are promoted wherever clinically and practically possible to enhance self-esteem and compliance.

P5 The play specialist discusses the goals of therapeutic play and ongoing observations with parents/carers.

OUTCOMES   O1 Children or young people identified by play specialists, parents or members of the multi-disciplinary team, as having increased anxieties are provided with additional support through planned therapeutic play activities.

O2 All the relevant professionals in the child's are kept informed.

O3 Parents/carers are informed of therapeutic play activities and outcomes.

O4 The plan, implementation and evaluation of therapeutic work is documented in the notes.

OUT-PATIENT SETTINGS

SUB TOPIC	**SAFEGUARDING CHILDREN**
CARE GROUP	Children and young people who attend the out-patient department
STANDARD	
OBJECTIVE	Observations of children at play and interacting with family members can contribute to child protection and social care.
RATIONALE	To ensure that children are able to communicate about anxiety provoking issues through play. This will be responded to appropriately.

Children's play and creative work reflects their internal and external life experiences and provides valuable insights into their worlds. A percentage of children visiting the out-patient department will have experienced abuse. They may reveal this consciously or unconsciously through play. Observation of the child at play provides an unobtrusive means to monitor and screen children. Play specialist observations contribute to the identification of children at risk and support the ongoing care of those already identified as at risk. Recognition of changes in behaviour of children who are regular attendees contributes to the assessment process.

STRUCTURES

S1 Play specialists attend training on child protection, local procedures and regular updates.

S2 The contribution of play specialists to child protection is recognised. Play specialists attend multi-professional meetings and have access to expert advice and extended study opportunities.

S3 Play specialists ensure all volunteers and students on placement have enhanced CRB clearance.

S4 Volunteer and student workers are given clear guidelines on local procedures for safe guarding children.

S5 Play staff, volunteer and student workers wear identification.

S6 Play specialists have access to clinical supervision and counselling when engaged in child protection work.

S7 Play specialists are involved in the recruitment and training of volunteers.

PROCESSES

P1 Play specialists screen for unusual interactions, themes and behaviours, whilst observing children at play on their own, with other children and/or family members.

P2 Formal assessments of developmental abilities, verbal and non- verbal interactions with family members are undertaken by the play specialists on referral from the multi-disciplinary team, for cases where there is a child protection concern.

PAEDIATRIC IN-PATIENTS

SUB TOPIC Cont.   **SAFEGUARDING CHILDREN**

PROCESSES   P3 Play specialists are involved in team discussions and are aware of reporting structures for child protection concerns.

P4 Play specialists use play and the relationship developed through it, to support anxious, distressed and/or disturbed children where there are child protection concerns.

P5 Play specialists take a proactive approach to maintaining professional boundaries by explaining the scope of their role and restricting social activity to that required for professional purposes. Patients are referred to the psychosocial support services where necessary.

P6 Play specialists undertake preparation work for internal physical examinations with consideration for the additional emotional stress involved for a child who has been sexually abused.

OUTCOMES   O1 Children's verbalised or played out communications are responded to appropriately.

O2 Disclosures of abuse or observations that cause concern are treated confidentially. Local policies for reporting are followed.

O3 Accurate, contemporaneous written records are completed to support child protection work.

O4 Where there are child protection concerns, drawings or writing produced by children are dated, timed and signed and stored in the notes,

O5 Social work and police investigations are supported in cases of alleged abuse.

SUB TOPIC   **SIBLING SUPPORT**

CARE GROUP   Siblings of children who are attending out-patient appointments

STANDARD

OBJECTIVE   To ensure that the siblings of patients attending out-patients appointments have access to play facilities and support.

RATIONALE   The play specialist in the out-patient department is well placed to observe and respond to sibling anxiety. The provision of play equipment and activities can make siblings feel welcome, encourages focused occupation and can reduce disruptive behaviour.

OUT-PATIENT SETTINGS

SUB TOPIC Cont.   **SIBLING SUPPORT**

STRUCTURES

S1 Parents/carers are notified if the out-patient play facilities are not supervised. They are reminded of their need to monitor safe play.

S2 Sufficient space and play equipment for siblings is provided.

S3 Sibling support is included in play specialist job descriptions and work plans.

S4 Play specialists have clear guidelines as to the action to be taken if siblings are left unattended in out-patient play areas.

PROCESSES

P1 Play specialists observe the play and interactions of siblings for signs of disturbance and misconceptions. Play specialists respond directly or indirectly to allow the expression of concerns and offer support.

P2 Play specialists encourage siblings to use the play facilities and participate in the activities provided.

P3 Play specialists communicate concerns about siblings with parents/carers.

OUTCOMES

O1 Siblings visiting the out-patient department are able to engage in play activities.

O2 Play specialist observations of siblings contribute to family centred care.

ACCIDENT AND EMERGENCY SETTINGS

SUB TOPIC	**CREATION AND MAINTENANCE OF AN AGE APPROPRIATE ENVIRONMENT**
CARE GROUP	All patients up to the age of 18 years old visiting the Accident and Emergency (A&E) department
STANDARD	
OBJECTIVE	To create and maintain an environment where children of all developmental abilities play safely. To ensure that distraction and alternative focus play equipment is available to all staff.
RATIONALE	Play is an essential part of childhood. Through play tension can be reduced. The provision of play equipment in the A&E department ensures that children feel welcome. It also encourages children to remain in one place thereby reducing potential conflicts with adult patients, traffic flow problems and the likelihood of unsafe play activity.
	Medical and nursing staff should have access to toys for distraction purposes, rewards and motivators.
STRUCTURES	S1 Purchases of distraction and play equipment take place after consultation between A&E staff and play specialists.
	S2 Cleaning and storage arrangements for play equipment are in accordance with infection control and risk management policies.
	S3 Play specialists receive training and guidance on infection control and risk management procedures.
	S4 A named person is responsible for inspecting the play equipment regularly.
	S5 Medical and nursing staff orientation programmes include information on the location of distraction equipment. Distraction techniques and the appropriate use of rewards and motivators are also covered.
	S6 Funding for distraction and play equipment forms part of the annual A&E budget.
	S7 Regular cleaning of toys takes place in line with local infection control policies.
PROCESSES	P1 Play specialists ensure play equipment is regularly inspected for damage or faults, removed and/or replaced if required.
	P2 Toys and games provided maintain interest during an average waiting time. These are culturally inclusive and appropriate for children of all developmental abilities.
	P3 Where play facilities are unsupervised; parents/carers are notified of their responsibility to supervise their children.

ACCIDENT AND EMERGENCY SETTINGS

SUB TOPIC Cont. **CREATION AND MAINTENANCE OF AN AGE APPROPRIATE ENVIRONMENT**

PROCESSES
P4 Play specialists ensure that the maintenance of distraction equipment takes places weekly and that stocks of reward incentives are maintained.

P5 All areas of the A&E department visited by children are equipped with toys and games.

P6 Ceilings and walls are decorated with interesting images, especially in areas where children are seen on trolleys.

OUTCOMES
O1 Children and their families feel welcome and use the play facilities provided.

O2 Play equipment does not deteriorate or date but is well maintained and renewed regularly.

O3 Medical, nursing staff and play specialists can access a range of distraction equipment at all times.

O4 The risks in designated play areas are minimised.

SUB TOPIC **PREPARATION FOR INVESTIGATIONS AND MEDICAL PROCEDURES**

CARE GROUP
All children over two years of age who are patients in the A&E department

STANDARD

OBJECTIVE
To enable patients to understand, at a developmentally appropriate level, the procedure they are to experience. The conditions for adaptive coping strategies are maximised. Patients are able to participate in the consent process.

RATIONALE
The sense of urgency, parental distress, and lack of time to assimilate new experiences and get to know staff can cause anxiety for children attending the Accident and Emergency department.

Research has demonstrated that preparation through play reduces anxiety, supports effective pain management and encourages co-operative behaviour.

STRUCTURES
S1 Training programmes for medical and nursing staff in A&E include sessions by play specialists which cover the evidence base for play preparation.

S2 The A&E department has mechanisms in place to ensure play specialists are informed of planned procedures.

S3 Play specialists undertake ongoing education to ensure excellence in preparation techniques. This includes reflective practice, peer review, professional conferences and local teaching sessions.

S4 New play specialists receive extensive orientation to the A&E department and observe all medical procedures.

ACCIDENT AND EMERGENCY SETTINGS

SUB TOPIC Cont.　　**PREPARATION FOR INVESTIGATIONS AND MEDICAL PROCEDURES**

PROCESSES　　P1 The play specialist assesses the developmental abilities and anxiety state of the patient prior to the preparation session.

P2 Parents/carers have the reasons for preparation and the approach to be taken explained to them.

P3 The play specialist engages the child in preparation play monitoring verbal and non-verbal communication throughout or explains procedures to the young person using suitable visual media to support learning.

P4 In emergency situations, information provided in preparation focuses on the essential details of the procedure and the behaviour required of the child.

P5 The play specialist halts preparation play if child shows undue anxiety and introduces a calming distraction activity.

P6 The play specialist acknowledges anxiety about pain and works collaboratively with staff and parents/carers to address concerns.

P7 The play specialist reports directly to child's nurse and documents the content and outcome of the preparation.

P8 Where possible, the play specialist returns to the patient to facilitate post-procedural mastery play and reinforcement of positive coping behaviours.

OUTCOMES　　O1 Age appropriate preparation for procedures, based on individual circumstances, is carried out prior to or during procedures.

O2 Parents/carers are encouraged to provide positive support to their child during procedures.

O3 The record of preparation is accessible to all health professionals involved with the child.

ACCIDENT AND EMERGENCY SETTINGS

SUB TOPIC   **DISTRACTION THERAPY AND ALTERNATIVE FOCUS ACTIVITIES**

CARE GROUP   All patients up to the age of 18 years old visiting the Accident and Emergency (A&E) department

STANDARD   STANDARD

OBJECTIVE   To help patients to cope with clinical procedures and investigations in the emergency setting by providing an alternative focus for their attention. To reduce the need for sedation or restraint. To contribute to the safe and accurate assessment and management of pain.

RATIONALE   Distraction therapy and alternative focus activities help children to cope with procedures by diverting their attention. Children are therefore less likely to be distressed and non-compliant, which creates a safer clinical environment. Children can gain confidence in themselves and those who care for them. As a result of the distraction therapy, the child may experience less pain.

In emergency situations, sedation involves risks and increases waiting times. Successful distraction therapy reduces the need for sedation.

STRUCTURES   S1 Play specialist hours of employment and staff ratios enable them to provide distraction therapy when required.

S2 The A&E department has mechanisms in place to ensure play specialists are informed of planned procedures.

S3 Play specialists undertake ongoing education to ensure excellence in distraction techniques.

S4 Funding is provided for distraction equipment.

S5 Play specialists lead training for department staff on distraction techniques, encouraging best practice.

S6 Visual distractions, in the form of projectors, posters, mobiles and wall stickers, are provided to support distraction therapy.

PROCESSES   P1 The play specialist gathers information about the procedure and establishes a plan in conjunction with the members of staff involved.

P2 For older children, the distraction techniques to be used are discussed and rehearsed prior to the event.

P3 Distraction techniques are discussed with the family and staff members involved.

ACCIDENT AND EMERGENCY SETTINGS

SUB TOPIC Cont.   **DISTRACTION THERAPY AND ALTERNATIVE FOCUS ACTIVITIES**

PROCESSES

P4 The play specialist praises achievements and positive coping behaviours and rewards with certificates and stickers, where appropriate.

P5 The play specialist records the distraction techniques and outcomes in the child's notes.

P6 The play specialist ensures that distraction equipment is readily available to all members of staff in the A&E department. Resources are restocked regularly.

OUTCOMES

O1 The number of Incidents of sedation and restraint is reduced due to the introduction of distraction during procedures.

O2 Patients are provided with age appropriate distraction during procedures, based on their individual circumstances.

O3 Parents/carers understand the purpose of and support the distraction therapy.

O4 A record of distraction techniques is accessible to all health professionals.

O5 Members of the A&E team are aware of the role of the play specialist with regard to distraction and request support for procedures.

SUB TOPIC   **GRIEF AND BEREAVEMENT SUPPORT**

CARE GROUP STANDARD

All patients up to 18 years old and family members attending the A&E department

OBJECTIVE

Play specialists use play and the relationship developed through it to informally and formally support children dealing with grief and bereavement issues.

RATIONALE

In an emergency situation, children will experience a range of emotions. If a sibling or parent is critically ill or dies, these will be accentuated. Support at is vital. The play specialist in A&E is well placed to provide age appropriate information and the opportunity for children to express their feelings.

STRUCTURES

S1 The play specialist team includes staff with considerable experience and training, who can lead and guide work on grief and bereavement issues.

S2 Play specialists have regular contact with members of the psychology team for clinical supervision for bereavement work.

S3 Play specialists attend regular multi-professional team meetings where bereavement work can be discussed and patients referred on if required.

S4 Play specialists have links with community support networks including health visitors and social workers.

ACCIDENT AND EMERGENCY SETTINGS

SUB TOPIC Cont.   **GRIEF AND BEREAVEMENT SUPPORT**

PROCESSES   P1 The play specialist is informed of critical care situations and prioritises siblings or offspring in this situation.

P2 The role of the play specialist is explained to parents/carers. The play specialist offers support for siblings.

P3 The play specialist acknowledges the significance of the child's feelings and uses play as a tool to explore issues around loss and grief and to correct any misconceptions.

P4 Calming play activities are used appropriately to maximise positive coping skills at a highly stressful time.

P5 The play specialist keeps parents/carers informed and documents interactions with siblings, contacting community support professionals where necessary.

OUTCOMES   O1 Therapeutic play and exploration of feelings are a part of the support provided to the young family members of a deceased or critically ill child or parent.

O2 Community health professionals are informed.

SUB TOPIC   **SAFEGUARDING CHILDREN**

CARE GROUP   All children & young people to the age of 18 years attending the A&E department

STANDARD

OBJECTIVE   To ensure the child protection needs of children and young people visiting the A&E department are identified and addressed.

To ensure that children are able to communicate anxieties through play and that this is responded to appropriately.

RATIONALE   The A&E department is an important point of contact between health professionals and children and young people. It provides a vital opportunity to identity children at risk. The observations of play specialists, conversations and interactions with children, young people and/or family members are an important part of the emergency team's screening process.

Children's play reflects their internal and external life experiences and provides valuable insights into their anxieties. Children in A&E may reveal upsetting experiences, either consciously or unconsciously through play.

ACCIDENT AND EMERGENCY SETTINGS

SUB TOPIC Cont. **SAFEGUARDING CHILDREN**

STRUCTURES

S1 Play specialists attend training on child protection, local procedures, and regular updates.

S2 The contribution of play specialists to child protection is recognised. Play specialists attend multi- professional meetings and have access to expert advice and extended study opportunities.

S3 Play specialists ensure all volunteer and student workers on placement have enhanced CRB clearance.

S4 Volunteer and student workers are given clear guidelines on local procedures for safe guarding children.

S5 Play specialists have access to clinical supervision and counselling when engaged in child protection work.

PROCESSES

P1 Observations of children at play and interacting with family members provide opportunities for the play specialist to screen for unusual interactions, themes and behaviours.

P2 The play specialist listens to children engaged in play and acknowledge anxieties expressed.

P3 The play specialist liaises with members of the A&E team where there are child protection concerns.

P4 The play specialist uses play and the relationship developed through it to support anxious and distressed children.

P5 Where there are child protection concerns, the play specialist in the A&E department works to establish a rapport with the young person involved.

P6 The play specialist recognises professional boundaries in child abuse cases.

P7 The play specialist undertakes preparation work for internal physical examinations with consideration for the additional emotional stress involved for a child, especially if he/she has been sexually abused.

OUTCOMES

O1 Children's verbalised or played out communications are responded to appropriately.

O2 The play specialist contributes to the screening of all children and young people entering the hospital.

O3 Disclosures of abuse and observations which suggest abuse, are treated confidentially. Local policies for reporting are followed.

ACCIDENT AND EMERGENCY SETTINGS

SUB TOPIC Cont. **SAFEGUARDING CHILDREN**

OUTCOMES
O4 Accurate, contemporaneous written records are completed to support child protection work.

O5 Where there are child protection concerns, drawings or writing produced by children are dated, timed and signed and stored in the child's notes.

O6 Social work and police investigations are supported in cases of alleged abuse.

SUB TOPIC **SIBLING SUPPORT**

CARE GROUP
Siblings of children and young people attending the A&E department

STANDARD

OBJECTIVE
To provide support for siblings in the emergency department.

RATIONALE
Children who accompany a sibling to the A&E department may become upset at a time when parental focus is on the sick or injured child. Siblings need play activities which will interest and calm them. Misconceptions about the cause of the illness or injury and medical interventions add to sibling distress. Sibling distress can be alleviated by the provision of suitable play activities and support.

STRUCTURES
S1 Staffing levels allow for the safe supervision of siblings in the A&E setting.

S2 Sufficient space and equipment is provided for siblings.

S3 Sibling support is part the play specialist job description and work plan.

PROCESSES
P1 The play specialist greets siblings and encourages them to use the play facilities.

P2 The play specialist observes sibling play and their interactions for signs of disturbance and/or misconceptions. The play specialist responds directly or indirectly to allow the expression of concerns and offers support.

P3 The play specialist helps siblings to understand what has happened and cope with their feelings.

P4 The play specialist records the numbers of siblings accessing the play service and the type of input provided. This data is collated and published periodically.

OUTCOMES
O1 Siblings visiting the A&E department are able to engage in play activities.

O2 Observations of sibling interactions contribute to family centred care.

O3 Where additional sibling work has taken place, there is liaison between key professionals in the child's life.

Accident and Emergency Settings

ACCIDENT AND EMERGENCY SETTINGS

SUB TOPIC Cont.   **SIBLING SUPPORT**

OUTCOMES   O4 Parents/carers feel supported whilst in the A&E department.

O5 Staff are able to deliver emergency care with minimum disruption from siblings.

O6 Data on siblings accessing the play service is available.

SUB TOPIC   **MOVING FROM ONE CLINICAL SETTING TO ANOTHER**

CARE GROUP   All patients up to the age of 18 and their families who are moving from A&E to ITU, assessment or in-patient units

STANDARD

OBJECTIVE   To reduce anxiety and uncertainty through the provision of age appropriate information. To acknowledging and address specific concerns. To handover information about the patient and family to play specialists and staff in the new setting.

RATIONALE   Any acute illness or injury which leads to a hospital admission has practical implications and raises anxiety levels. Play specialists in the Accident and Emergency department are well placed to anticipate issues that will be of concern to the family. These can be addressed through the provision of information and support. Written details of successful preparation methods, distraction techniques, and play and developmental assessments ensure continuity of care. A seamless transition is appreciated by patients and staff.

STRUCTURES   S1 The orientation programme of A&E play specialists includes meetings with the staff in the Intensive Care Unit, admissions wards and assessment units.

S2 Professional networks between play specialists are maintained through joint meetings, training and shared projects.

S3 Staffing levels in A&E enable play specialists to develop a range of materials to prepare patients and their families for a transfer.

S4 Mechanisms exist for the translation of information into languages reflecting the ethnicity of the local population.

ACCIDENT AND EMERGENCY SETTINGS

SUB TOPIC Cont.   **MOVING FROM ONE CLINICAL SETTING TO ANOTHER**

PROCESSES

P1 Play specialists are informed about arrangements for transfer to other clinical settings.

P2 Play specialists use photographs, film media and other visual aids to provide age appropriate information to patients prior to the transfer.

P3 Preparation information includes information about the staff and care they will receive on the new unit.

P4 The Information provided is adapted to recognise the emotional and physical state of the patient and family.

OUTCOMES

O1 Patients being transferred from the A&E department are provided with sufficient age appropriate information about their destination.

O2 Practical information for parents/carers is provided prior to transfer from the A&E Department.

O3 Patient anxieties are acknowledged and managed through play and discussion.

O4 Staff admitting patients from A&E are given information about successful distraction and preparation interventions, and assessments.

COMMUNITY SETTINGS

SUB TOPIC — **PROVISION OF RECREATIONAL AND THERAPEUTIC ACTIVITIES**

CARE GROUP — Hospital or hospice patients who receive out-patient or palliative care at home.

STANDARD

OBJECTIVE — To provide play activities to help a child or young person meet identified social, emotional or developmental goals. To contribute to medical or nursing care plans.

RATIONALE — Children who are seriously ill, physically restricted or awaiting surgery can benefit from supervised therapeutic play sessions in their own home. Play facilitates communication and the development of coping strategies.

In some cases, play specialists who are hospital based, visit children in their homes, providing continuity and liaison between settings.

Play specialists can be employed as part of community nursing teams and in hospices.

STRUCTURES

S1 There are sufficient play specialists to ensure all community patients who require play sessions receive them.

S2 Sufficient space is allocated for the safe storage of play equipment for community work.

S3 Play specialists attend regular multi-professional meetings.

S4 Care plans include contributions from play specialists.

S5 Sufficient funds are provided to purchase and renew safe and appropriate toys, games, craft materials and play equipment for children with special needs.

S6 Clear written referral criteria for the play service are provided to local community and hospital teams.

S7 Information about the home setting is available to play specialists Play specialists are informed if a child is on the At Risk Register.

S8 There is an established system of booking out and in before and after home visits. Risk management procedures are followed.

PROCESSES

P1 The play specialist makes an appointment for a home visit with the family. This visit minimises disruption to the child's normal routine, whilst maximising the likelihood of engagement and attention.

P2 The play specialist establishes clear objectives with new patients and their parents/carers.

SUB TOPIC Cont. **PROVISION OF RECREATIONAL AND THERAPEUTIC ACTIVITIES**

PROCESSES

P3 The play specialist assesses the needs, abilities and interests of the patient and sets short and long-term goals.

P4 The play specialist liaises with the multi-disciplinary team and family to arrange play sessions.

P5 The play specialist observes and assesses verbal and non-verbal communication during free and directed play sessions. Assessment, implementation and evaluation of play programme goals takes place.

P6 Direction, interaction and support are provided through play. A variety of sensory stimulation and play activities are provided.

P7 Parents/carers are encouraged to join in with play activities, where appropriate. They are informed of play specialist assessments and plans.

P8 The play specialist ensures issues identified are documented and shared with key professionals in the child's life.

OUTCOMES

O1 Children who are referred to the community play specialist are provided with a wide range of play activities which stimulate sensory, cognitive and social pathways.

O2 Parents/carers are supported in providing suitable play opportunities.

O3 Play opportunities which meet the patient's identified developmental, adaptation and emotional needs are provided.

O4 Patients and their families are aware of the role of the play specialist, play service hours and the importance of play.

O5 The risks associated with working in the community are actively managed and minimised.

COMMUNITY SETTINGS

SUB TOPIC	**INFORMATION ABOUT HOSPITALS**
CARE GROUP	Individuals and groups in the community requiring information about hospitals or medical conditions.
STANDARD	
OBJECTIVE	To provide accessible and meaningful information to children and their families. To acknowledge the variety of emotional responses to hospital experiences.
RATIONALE	Play specialists are often asked to provide talks and/or visits to groups or individuals in the community. A school where there is a sick child returning to school after a long illness or where education about hospitals is part of the curriculum may request play specialist input.

Children are prone to misconceptions and anxieties about hospitals and ill health. They need age appropriate information that is designed specifically for them. With such information, children are equipped to better cope with hospital experiences and provide peer support. |
| STRUCTURES | S1 Play specialists undertake training in presentation skill. Play specialist are provided with opportunities to learn about medical conditions and community issues.

S2 Clear criteria for community presentations are established between play specialists and line managers. These include fee charging criteria.

S3 Play specialists have adequate time, space and equipment to prepare for presentations.

S4 Play specialists establish and maintain professional networks within community education, nursing and social services. |
| PROCESSES | P1 The play specialist establishes clear objectives for presentations or information sharing sessions, based on knowledge gathered from those involved.

P2 The play specialist allows time to prepare information to be presented and gather visual materials.

P3 The play specialist notes verbal and non-verbal anxiety cues in the audience and assesses options for managing these, alerting local adults or professionals where appropriate. |
| OUTCOMES | O1 Age appropriate information provided by play specialists enables children to cope with their own hospital experiences and those of others.

O2 Play specialists adopt an inclusive approach which enables liaison between community and hospital services.

O3 Fund raising efforts for play and community nursing services are supported through good quality presentations. |

COMMUNITY SETTINGS

SUB TOPIC **PREPARATION FOR INVESTIGATIONS, SURGERY AND MEDICAL PROCEDURES**

CARE GROUP Children over two years of age who require preparation in home setting

STANDARD

OBJECTIVE To ensure that paediatric patients are able to understand, at a developmentally appropriate level, the procedure they are to experience.

To ensure that the conditions for developing adaptive coping strategies are maximised.

RATIONALE A child centred approach to information giving is vital. Research has demonstrated that preparation through play reduces stress and encourages compliance. This may also reduce a child's experience of pain. For children with extreme anxiety or additional problems, preparation in a community setting is appropriate.

STRUCTURES S1 Play specialist hours enable them to assess, plan and implement preparation programmes in the community when required.

S2 Community and hospital teams are informed of the role of the community play specialist and are aware of the referral criteria for children requiring preparation.

S3 Community play specialists undertake ongoing education to ensure excellence in preparation techniques. This includes reflective practice, peer review, professional conferences and local teaching.

S4 The orientation programme for community play specialists includes visits to local hospitals and treatment centres.

S5 Community play specialists establish and maintain professional networks within community and hospital teams.

PROCESSES P1 Parents/carers have the reasons for preparation and the approach to be taken explained to them.

P2 The play specialist gathers information about the patient requiring preparation through observation and interaction with the child and dialogue with family and staff members.

P3 The play specialist recognises the child's psychological responses to learning. The play specialist provides verbal information and uses visual aids.

P4 The play specialist engages the child in preparation play monitoring verbal and non-verbal communication throughout, in one or more sessions.

P5 The play specialist ceases preparation play if child shows undue anxiety. The possible reasons for anxiety are explored at an appropriate time.

COMMUNITY SETTINGS

SUB TOPIC Cont.	**PREPARATION FOR INVESTIGATIONS, SURGERY AND MEDICAL PROCEDURES**
PROCESSES	P6 The play specialist acknowledges anxiety about pain and works collaboratively with staff and parents/carers to address concerns.
	P7 The play specialist informs parents/carers of the outcomes of the play preparation, encouraging the rehearsal and use of coping strategies.
	P8 The play specialist reports directly to the community and in-patient medical and nursing teams and documents the content and outcome of the preparation in the child's notes.
	P9 The play specialist returns to the patient's home to facilitate post-procedural mastery play and debriefing.
OUTCOMES	O1 Age appropriate preparation for procedures, based on the individual child's circumstances, is carried out in a timely fashion.
	O2 Parents/carers are informed of the purpose, content and outcome of preparation.
	O3 The preparation record is accessible to all health professionals involved with the child.
	O4 The opportunities for a child to cope well with procedures or surgery are maximised. There is liaison between community and hospital staff.
	O5 The play specialist refers children who do not show reduced anxiety after an appropriate number of structured preparation sessions back to the referring consultant.
SUB TOPIC	**THERAPEUTIC PLAY ACTIVITIES**
CARE GROUP	Children over 2 years of age where there is defined concern
STANDARD	
OBJECTIVE	Issues which arise as a result of hospital experiences, illness or treatment are identified and responded to using a range of age appropriate therapeutic techniques
RATIONALE	Illness and/or hospital experiences in childhood may cause short or long term psychological harm. This can impact on adaptation to home life following hospital admissions and on ongoing medical and nursing care. Children who are identified as having increased anxieties are provided with additional support through therapeutic play sessions.

COMMUNITY SETTINGS

SUB TOPIC Cont.   **THERAPEUTIC PLAY ACTIVITIES**

STRUCTURES

S1 Community and hospital teams are informed of the role of the community play specialist in supporting children with persistent adaptation problems following medical interventions and/or illness.

S2 Local referral criteria for therapeutic play sessions with a play specialist exist.

S3 Liaison between play specialists, medical and nursing staff ensures accurate information is gathered and joint planning of therapeutic interventions takes place.

S4 Play specialists undertake ongoing education to ensure competency in therapeutic play work. This includes reflective practice and clinical supervision.

PROCESSES

P1 The play specialist explains the aims of the visit and the approach to be taken to parents/carers, establishing a collaborative approach.

P2 The play specialist uses both familiar and hospital play activities to establish a relationship with the child. During the play session, the play specialist observes and assesses verbal and non-verbal communication for atypical behaviour, or concerns.

P3 Therapeutic play interventions are planned, implemented and evaluated within one or more home visits.

P4 A variety of materials and approaches are used. Sensory stimulation is used initiate the exploration of anxieties, mastery play and the resolution of issues related to the hospital experience or illness.

P5 The play specialist ensures that the issues identified are documented and shared with key professionals in the child's life.

OUTCOMES

O1 Parents/carers are informed of the purpose and outcome of therapeutic play activities.

O2 Children identified as having increased anxieties by the play specialist, parents/carers or members of the multi-disciplinary team are provided with additional support through planned therapeutic play activities.

O3 All relevant professionals in the patient's life are kept informed.

O4 The play specialist refers children who do not show reduced anxiety after several therapeutic play sessions back to the referring consultant.

COMMUNITY SETTINGS

SUB TOPIC | **SUPPORT FOR GRIEF AND BEREAVEMENT ISSUES**

CARE GROUP Terminally ill children and their families. Children who have recently experienced a major loss. Children dealing with losses associated with illness and/or major injury.

STANDARD

OBJECTIVE Play specialists use play activities and the relationship developed through them, to support children dealing with grief and bereavement issues.

RATIONALE Play is a channel for communication, and a means of learning to understand and manage difficult issues. Play specialists use play to actively support terminally ill children or those experiencing a major loss.

STRUCTURES S1 Community and hospital teams are informed of the role of the community play specialist in supporting children with bereavement issues.

S2 Clear referral criteria for bereavement work with the play specialist are established locally.

S3 Play specialists undertake ongoing education to ensure competency in working with childhood bereavement.

S4 The orientation programme for play specialists includes visits to local hospitals and hospices.

S5 Play specialists establish and maintain professional networks in the community and adult and children's hospice teams.

S6 Play specialists have clinical supervision for bereavement work.

S7 Play specialists attend regular multi-professional team meetings where bereavement work can be discussed and patients referred on if required.

PROCESSES P1 The play specialist explains the aims of the visit and the approach to be taken to parents/carers, establishing a collaborative approach.

P2 The play specialist uses familiar play activities to establish a relationship with the child. During the play session, the play specialist observes and assesses verbal and non-verbal communication noting issues to do with grief and loss.

P3 The play specialist acknowledges the significance of the child's feelings and uses play as a tool to explore issues around and correct misconceptions about loss and grief.

COMMUNITY SETTINGS

SUB TOPIC Cont. **SUPPORT FOR GRIEF AND BEREAVEMENT ISSUES**

PROCESSES

P4 A variety of materials and approaches are used. Both free and directed play activities allow child-led as well as adult-led exploration of issues related to bereavement and loss.

P5 The play specialist documents identified issues and ongoing work and shares relevant information with the key professionals in the child's life.

P6 The play specialist discusses the play interventions and ongoing observations with parents/carers.

P7 The play specialist maintains his/her knowledge of national organisations, websites and literature to support bereavement work.

OUTCOMES

O1 Play interventions to address bereavement issues for identified children are planned, implemented and evaluated.

O2 All relevant professionals in the child's life are kept informed.

O3 Parents/carers are informed and enabled to support their child.

O4 Where additional needs are identified, the child is referred to the Child and Adolescent Mental Health Service (CAMHS) or other appropriate professional.

SUB TOPIC **SAFEGUARDING CHILDREN**

CARE GROUP

All children & young people up to the age of 18 seen by the play specialist in the community

STANDARD

OBJECTIVE

To ensure that the child protection needs of children and young people seen by the play specialist in the community are identified and addressed.

To ensure that children are able to communicate anxieties through play and that this is responded to appropriately.

RATIONALE

Play specialist community sessions provide an important point of contact and a vital opportunity to identity children at risk. The observations of play specialists, conversations and interactions with children, young people and/or family members are an important part of the community team's screening process.

Children's play reflects their internal and external life experiences and provides valuable insights into their anxieties. Children at home may reveal upsetting experiences, consciously or unconsciously, through play.

COMMUNITY SETTINGS

SUB TOPIC Cont.	**SAFEGUARDING CHILDREN**

STRUCTURES

S1 Play specialists attend child protection training which includes local procedures. Play specialists attend regular child protection updates.

S2 The contribution of play specialists to child protection is recognised. Play specialists attend multi-professional meetings and have access to expert advice and extended study opportunities.

S3 Play specialists are provided with clear guidance for working with children and families in their homes.

S4 Play specialists have access to clinical supervision and counselling when engaged in child protection work.

PROCESSES

P1 Observations of children at play and interacting with family members provide opportunities for the play specialist to screen for unusual interactions, themes and behaviours.

P2 Play specialists listen to children engaged in play and acknowledge anxieties expressed.

P3 Play specialists liaise closely with members of the child's health and social care team about child protection concerns.

P4 Play specialists take a proactive approach to maintaining professional boundaries by ensuring that children understand the scope of their role, restricting social activity to that required for professional purposes and referring patients to the psychosocial support services where necessary.

P5 Play specialists recognise professional boundaries in child abuse cases.

OUTCOMES

O1 Children's verbalised or played out communications are heard and responded to appropriately.

O2 Play specialists contribute to the screening process for children and young people at risk.

O3 Disclosures of abuse and observations that suggest abuse are treated confidentially. Local policies for reporting are followed.

O4 Accurate, contemporaneous written records are completed to support child protection work.

O5 Where there are child protection concerns, drawings or writing produced by the child are dated, timed and signed and stored in the notes.

O6 Social work and police investigations are supported in cases of alleged abuse.

SECTION

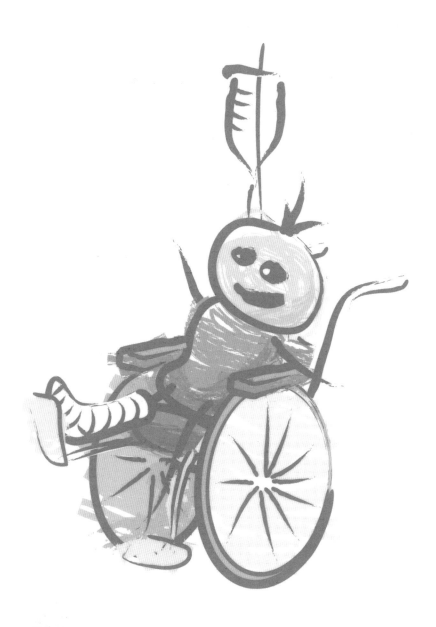

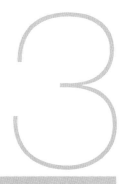

3

THREE

References

References

1. Nightingale, F. (1872) Address from Ms Nightingale to the probationer nurses in the "Nightingale Fund" School at St Thomas' Hospital.

2. Hogg, C. (1990) "Quality Management for Children: Play in Hospital." Play in Hospital Liaison Committee

3. Department of Health. (2003) Getting the Right Start: The National Service Framework for Children, Young People and Maternity Services. Hospital Standard.

4. Department of Health. (2003) Every Child Matters.

5. Donabedian Avedis. (2003) "An Introduction to Quality Assurance in Health Care," O.U.P.

6. Harvey S, Hales-Tooke, (1972)" Play in Hospital", Faber and Faber.

7. DHSS. (1976) "Report of the Expert Group on Play for Children in Hospital", (HC(76)5).

8. Save the Children Fund. (1989) "Hospital: A Deprived Environment for Children?"

9. Department of Health. (1993) "Welfare of Children and Young People in Hospital".

10. Audit Commission Review 'Children First' (A Study of Hospital Services) HMSO, London

11. Department of Health (1995) "The Patients' Charter Services for Children and Young People" HMSO, London

12. Ministry of Health HMSO (1959) The Platt Report "The Welfare of Children in Hospital"

13. United Nations. "Convention for the Rights of the Child" 1989 (ratified by the UK Government in 1991)

14. Schwartz BH et al (1983) Effects of psychological preparation on children hospitalised for dental operations Journal of Pediatrics 1983

15. Sylva K and Stein A (1990) "Effects of hospitalisation on young children" Child Psychology and Psychiatry Vol 12

16. Sylva, K. (1993) "Play in Hospital: When and Why It's Effective" Current Paediatrics 3.

17. Visintainer MA Wolfer JA (1975) "Psychological Preparation for surgical paediatric patients: The effect on children's and parent's stress responses" Pediatrics 56 187-202

18. Melamed BG Siegel LJ (1975) "Reduction of anxiety in children' facing hospitalisation and surgery by use of filmed modelling" J Consulting Clinical Psychology 43:511-521664

19. Rodin J (1983) "Will this hurt?" London RCN

20. Duff, A.J.A. (2003) "Incorporating psychological processes into routine paediatric venepuncture" Archives of Diseases in Childhood Vol 88 Iss 10pp

21. Varni, J,W et al (1995) "Management of Pain and Distress". In M Roberts (Ed) Handbook of Paediatric Psychology

22. Peterson, L & Shigeomi, C (1982) "One year follow up of elective surgery; child patients receiving pre-operative preparation" Journal of Pediatric Psychology 7 Vol 43–48

23. Eckhardt LO & Prugh DG (1978) "Preparing children for psychologically painful medical and surgical procedures" In Psychosocial Aspects of Pediatric Care Ed. E Gellert. Grune & Stratton

24. Ferguson BF (1979) "Preparing young children for hospitalisation; a comparison of two methods" Pediatrics 64: 656–664

25. Petrillo M (1972) "Preparing children and parents for hospitalisation and treatment" Pediatric Annuals 1(3) 24–41

26. Frued, A. (1952) "The role of Bodily Illness in the Mental Life of Children" Psychoanalytic Study of the Child.

27. Tisza, VB. et al (1970) "The use of a play programme by hospitalised children." Journal of American Child Psychiatry Vol 9, pt 3, pp 513–531.

28. Caines, E. (1992) NHS Management Executive Letter EL(92)42 Department of Health, July.

Source materials

Barnard, S. Hartigan, G. (1998) "Clinical Audit in Physiotherapy; From Theory into Practice" Butterworth-Heinemann.

Morrell, C. Harvey, G. (1999) "The Clinical Audit Handbook; Improving the Quality of Health Care" Balliere Tindall RCN.

Lugon, M, Secker-Walker, J, Eds (1999) "Clinical Governance; Making it Happen" RSM

Rogoff, B. (2003) "The Cultural Nature of Human Development" OUP.

Official Documents of the Children Life Council of America (2002).

Official Documents of the Hospital Play Specialist Association of Aotearoa /New Zealand Inc. (2004)

Department of Health. (1993) Clinical Audit ; Meeting and Improving Standards in Healthcare, HMSO London.

Guidance and Units: Edexcel Level 4 Professional Development Diploma in Specialised Play for Sick Children and Young People, July 2004.

Clinical Practice Guidelines; The recognition and assessment of acute pain in children; Implementation Guide RCN March 2001 ISBN 1873853 99 8.

List of professionals consulted

The following people reviewed and commented on the first draft of the publication. Their support is much appreciated.

Charlotte Bramley	Hospital play specialist	Kaleidoscope Kensington and Chelsea
Elaine Eastman	Play services manager	Bristol Royal Hospital for Children
Gill Caddy	Play co-ordinator	Royal Cornwall Hospital
Norma Jun-Tai	Play co-ordinator	Kingston Hospital Surrey
Jean Wilde	Retired hospital play specialist & play therapist	
Carol Page	Hospital play specialist	Wycombe General Hospital
Susan Fairclough	Play services manager	Manchester Children's Hospital
Jill Vines	Play services manager	Glasgow Children's Hospital
Karen Kelly	Play services manager	Birmingham Children's Hospital NHS Trust
Suzanne Storer	Chairman	Hospital Play Staff Education Trust
Peg Belson MBE	NAHPS Patron	
Jackie Broadhurst	Hospital play specialist	Withybush General Hospital
Steve Andrews	Charge nurse	University College Hospitals NHS Foundation Trust
Frances Binns	Therapeutic & specialised play consultant	Manchester Children's Hospitals
Christine Baines	Hospital play specialist	Addenbrookes Hospital Cambridge
Angela White	Hospital play specialist	Addenbrookes Hospital Cambridge
Nic Phillips	Hospital play specialist	North Hampshire Hospital
Sue Simpson	Hospital play specialist	University Hospital of Wales
Ishbel Proctor	Play co-ordinator	Royal Hospital for Sick Children Edinburgh
Sian Hulbert	Hospital play specialist	University Hospital of Wales
Tracey Roe	Play services manager	The Royal London Hospital
Miriam Sincliar	Hospital play specialist	Leicester Royal Infirmary
Richard Wilson	Paediatrician, NAHPS Patron	Royal College of Paediatrics and Child Health
Beverly Boyd		Royal College of Nursing
Sandra Dumitrescu	Hospital play specialist	Ty Hafan Children's Hospice

Location of Audit	Sunshine Regional Health Authority
Purpose of Audit	The Sunshine Region Play Specialist Group want to lobby for better clinical supervision after the nervous breakdown of one of its members
Audit topic	Paediatric In-patients Directed therapeutic play activities Structures 1, 3 and 4
Method chosen	Questionnaire to 40 named play specialists in region
Who is involved?	Sunshine Region Play Specialist Group

Example of a Postal Questionnaire

Please give salary/grade

STRUCTURE OUTCOME

S1 The play specialist team includes staff with considerable experience who can lead and guide therapeutic play

Q How many years have you been practising as a Hospital Play Specialist?

S3 Play specialists have regular contact with members of the psychology team for clinical supervision of therapeutic work.

Q How many times in the past 12 months have you met with your line manager for one to one discussions?

Q How many times in the past 12 months have you had group or individual clinical supervision?

Q How many times in the past 12 months have you had the opportunity to attend an event for professional development purposes (eg workplace case discussion groups, seminars, conferences, professional courses other than mandatory courses i.e. fire safety)

EXAMPLE ONE cont.

S4 Play specialists attend regular multi-professional team meetings where therapeutic work can be discussed and patients referred on if required.

Q How often do you attend multi professional team meetings?

Q Can you ask psychologists, psychotherapists, social workers, or other members of the multi-disciplinary team to review a patient you have worked with?

Q How often do you do this?

Any other comments?

Location of Audit	Ward 4B
Purpose of Audit	To assess and improve the quality of individual play specialists work as part of the performance management policy
Audit topic	Paediatric In-patients
	Preparation for tests, surgery and other procedures
	Processes P1, P2, P3, P4, P5, P6, P7, P8, P9.
Method chosen	Observation and discussion
Who is involved?	Play co-ordinator, sister, play specialist

The play co-ordinator explains the purpose of the observation to the play specialist and local management team. A target number of preparation sessions to be observed is set. The criteria for the observation are set using the processes described in this sub topic.

PROCESS OUTCOME	OBSERVATION QUESTIONS
P1 Play specialists gather information about the patient requiring preparation through observation and interaction with the child and dialogue with family and staff.	What information is obtained prior to the preparation session?
P2 Parents/carers have the reasons for preparation and the approach to be taken explained to them.	Are adult carers given appropriate explanations?
P3 The play specialist assesses the child's psychological responses to learning. The play specialist provides verbal information and uses visual aids to prepare the child.	What visual aids are used? What evidence is there of recognition of child's psychological response to the play preparation session?
P4 The play specialist engages the child in preparation play monitoring verbal and non-verbal communication throughout, in one or more sessions.	Are verbal and non-verbal cues noted by play specialist? How?

EXAMPLE TWO cont.

PROCESS OUTCOME	OBSERVATION QUESTIONS
P5 The play specialist halts preparation play if child shows undue anxiety and explores the possible reasons for this anxiety at an appropriate time.	Does the play specialist respond to non verbal and verbal anxiety cues?
P6 The play specialist acknowledges anxiety about pain and works collaboratively with staff and carers to address the child's concerns.	Are worries about pain discussed? Are methods of pain relief mentioned?
P7 The play specialist informs parents/carers of the outcomes of the play preparation and the coping strategies identified.	Does the play specialist report back to parents, encouraging the use of coping strategies?
P8 The play specialist reports directly to patient's nurse and documents the content and outcome of the preparation.	Assess content of written documentation
P9 The play specialist returns to the patient to facilitate post procedural mastery play and debriefing.	Does the play specialist return to the patient to facilitate post procedural mastery play and debriefing?

Location of Audit	Seaside Hospital Trust
Purpose of Audit	To improve quality of distraction play and alternative focus activities throughout the hospital
Audit topic	Outcome measures for each distraction and alternative focus sub topic in A&E, Paediatric In-patients and Out-patients
Method chosen	Single day audit; play specialists take it in turns to attend each others' wards to assess outcomes on that day
Who is involved?	All play specialists in Trust, representatives from nursing and medical staff across Trust, Modern Matron, patients and their families

OUTCOMES	AUDIT QUESTIONS
O1 Age appropriate distraction during procedures, based on individual child's circumstances, is carried out in a timely fashion.	How many times does the play specialist provide distraction activities?
	How much time does each episode take?
	How often was the play specialist asked to carry out distraction?
	How often did the play specialist identify children who needed distraction?
O2 Parents/carers understand the purpose and support the process of distraction.	Does the play specialist address the parent/carers and explain purpose of the distraction?
O3 The record of distraction activities is accessible to all health professionals involved with the child.	How many times does the play specialist record the distraction activity so that it is accessible to health professionals in other settings?